W. Meyer

Monoclonal Antibodies

The Basics

Series Advisors:

Rob Beynon UMIST, Manchester, UK
Chris Howe Department of Biochemistry, University of Cambridge, Cambridge, UK

Monoclonal Antibodies

Forthcoming titles

PCR
Biological Centrifugation
Separating Cells
Analysing Chromosomes
Gene Mapping
Reconstructing Molecular Evolutionary Trees

Monoclonal Antibodies

Preparation and use of monoclonal antibodies and engineered antibody derivatives

Edited by

Heddy Zola PhD

Child Health Research Institute, Women's and Children's Hospital, Adelaide, Department of Paediatrics, University of Adelaide, Department of Paediatrics, Flinders University, and Co-operative Research Centre for Diagnostic Technologies, Australia

BIOS

Springer

H. Zola
Child Health Research Institute, Women's and Children's Hospital, Adelaide, Department of Paediatrics, University of Adelaide, Department of Paediatrics, Flinders University, and Co-operative Research Centre for Diagnostic Technologies, Australia

---

Published in the United States of America, its dependent territories and Canada by arrangement with BIOS Scientific Publishers Ltd, 9 Newtec Place, Magdalen Road, Oxford OX4 1RE, UK

A CIP catalogue record for this book is available from the British Library.

ISBN 0-387-91590-7 Springer-Verlag New York Berlin Heidelberg SPIN 10738095

Springer-Verlag New York Inc.
175 Fifth Avenue, New York
NY 10010–7858, USA

Production Editor: Fran Kingston
Typeset by Creative Associates, Oxford, UK
Printed by TJ International, Padstow, Cornwall, UK

The Basics

Contents

Contributors ix
Preface xi
Glossary xiii

Chapter 1 Antibodies as laboratory and therapeutic reagents 1

H Zola

1. Introduction: antibody specificity and diversity 1
2. Antibody specificity: protein structure 2
3. The immunoglobulin constant region: form and functions 3
4. The cells that make antibody 5
5. The basis of antibody specificity and diversity: unique genetic mechanisms 6
6. Polyclonal antisera 8
7. Monoclonal antibodies 9
8. The major differences between monoclonal and polyclonal antibodies 10
9. Applications of antibodies in the laboratory 12
10. Therapeutic applications of antibodies 13
11. Improving on nature – antibody engineering 15
12. Replacing nature – antibodies from gene libraries 15
13. Conclusions 15

Chapter 2 Hybridoma technology: making monoclonal antibodies 17

B Hunt, H Zola and C Goddard

1. Introduction 17
2. Theoretical basis 17
3. Cell culture 17
4. Screening assay 20
5. Immunization 21
6. Myeloma cells 23
7. Fusion protocol 24
8. Post-fusion care 24
9. Cloning 26
10. Cryopreservation 26
11. Specificity and isotyping 26

12. Mycoplasma 27
13. Large scale antibody production 27
14. Antibody purification 29
15. Storage and quality control 30
Protocol 2.1: Screening hybridomas by enzyme-linked immunoassay (ELISA) 32
Protocol 2.2: Conjugation of antigen to a carrier protein 34
Protocol 2.3: Immunization with a soluble protein available in quantity 35
Protocol 2.4: Fusion – standard protocol using polyethylene glycol (PEG) 36
Protocol 2.5: Cloning of hybridoma cells 39
Protocol 2.6: Cryopreservation of hybridoma cells 40
Protocol 2.7: Purification of IgG1 on Protein G 42

Chapter 3 Antibody engineering 45

MA Thiel, G Pilkington and H Zola

1. Introduction 45
2. Choice of antibody designs to suit specific applications 46
3. Chimeric and humanized whole antibodies 51
4. Single domain antigen binding fragments 52
5. Engineering antibody fragments 53
6. Expression of antibody fragments 55
7. Purification of scFv antibody fragments 57
8. Phage display 57
Protocol 3.1: Preparation and selection of phage display library of Fab fragments 67
Protocol 3.2: Purification of human Fab 79

Chapter 4 Applications of monoclonal antibodies to the study of molecules in solution 81

DA Brooks

1. Introduction 81
2. ELISA (enzyme linked immuno-adsorbent assay) 83
3. Protein epitope delineation 86
4. Assays of antibody-bound antigen 87
5. Immunoaffinity chromatography 89
6. Western blotting 91
7. Immunoprecipitation and radiolabel synthesis/processing 92
8. Immuno-organelle binding assays 93
Protocol 4.1: Immunoaffinity chromatography 95
Protocol 4.2: Western blotting 97
Protocol 4.3: Radiolabel-immunoprecipitation protocol 99

Chapter 5 Applications of monoclonal antibodies in microbiology **101**

T Kok, P Li and I Gardner

1. Introduction 101
2. Diagnosing infection 102
3. Viruses 104
4. Mycoplasma and chlamydia 108
5. Applications in bacteriology 110
6. Parasitic and fungal infections 121

Protocol 5.1: Detection of *Neisseria meningitidis* antigen by agglutination of monoclonal antibody-coated latex particles 124

Chapter 6 Applications of monoclonal antibodies to the study of cells and tissues **127**

H Zola

1. Introduction 127
2. The complexity of cells: the human CD antigens illustrate the heterogeneity of cellular composition 128
3. Cell markers: identification and enumeration of specific cell types 130
4. Antibody-based cell separation 139
5. Antibody-based cell destruction or agglutination 141
6. Analysis of function 141
7. Tissue analysis 142

Protocol 6.1: Direct immunofluorescence 144

Index 147

The Basics

Contributors

DA Brooks, Department of Chemical Pathology, Women's and Children's Hospital, Adelaide, Australia.

I Gardner, Department of Immunology, Queensland Medical Laboratories, Brisbane, Australia.

C Goddard, Co-operative Research Centre for Tissue Growth and Repair, and Gropep Pty Ltd, Adelaide, Australia.

B Hunt, Co-operative Research Centre for Tissue Growth and Repair, and Gropep Pty Ltd, Adelaide, Australia.

T Kok, Department of Microbiology, University of Adelaide, Australia.

P Li, Department of Microbiology, University of Adelaide, Australia.

G Pilkington, Intracel Corporation, 1330 Piccard Drive, Rockville, MD, USA.

MA Thiel, Department of Ophthalmology, Flinders University, and Child Health Research Institute, South Australia.

The Basics

Preface

Monoclonal antibodies have revolutionized many aspects of biology and medicine since their first description in 1976. There is now an extensive literature describing the preparation and application of monoclonal antibodies, including two previous books by the principal author of this book. Why do we need another one?

There are two major reasons. The first is that monoclonal antibodies are poised to break new ground, as therapeutic agents. Until now the lack of success, with one major exception, of monoclonal antibodies as therapeutic agents has stood in sharp contrast with their success as laboratory reagents. The second reason is that monoclonal antibodies have been around for a generation, long enough to be taken for granted. Scientists who worked with antibodies through the 1980s understand the profound differences in specificity, reproducibility and analytical power between monoclonal antibodies and conventional, polyclonal, antisera. That generation of scientists is being replaced by a new generation, scientists very much at home with genetic techniques, but with little feeling for or interest in the different types of antibody they may need to use. Yet an understanding of antibodies is necessary for their most effective use, and genetically manipulated antibody-based molecules are coming back to the fore. A substantial proportion of therapeutic substances under clinical trial at present are antibodies or their derivatives.

This book is directed primarily at the new generation, new research workers in biological and medical research, including PhD students. Experienced researchers whose expertise is not primarily with antibody-based techniques, but who need to apply antibodies in their research, may have the same unfamiliarity with the special properties of monoclonal antibodies (not all good) and this book is also intended for them.

The book begins with a discussion of the antibody molecule, its structural features, the genetic mechanisms that lead to the unique diversity and specificity of antibodies, and the biology of the B cells that make antibodies. This material is not usually described in any detail in books on antibody technology, but it is interesting, and knowledge of the underlying biology may just give the scientist making or using antibodies an unfair advantage over competitors. The book describes the preparation of monoclonal antibodies and their genetically engineered derivatives, and the major uses of these reagents. Preparation of polyclonal antibodies is not covered, to keep the book focused. The differences between monoclonal antibodies and polyclonal antisera are stressed, as are the consequent differences in techniques required to get the best results from monoclonal and polyclonal antibodies.

In keeping with the rest of the series, the book presents experimental details for key methods. However, the field is too large to provide full protocols for all relevant methods. To keep the book to manageable size, common techniques which are not specifically associated with antibody techniques are not described – techniques such as polyacrylamide gel electrophoresis, column chromatography. Where appropriate, references are given to other manuals. Techniques which are central to monoclonal antibodies, in particular hybridization, cloning, etc., are described in detail. For each method, a recommended procedure is described, together with discussion of variations on the basic method and the circumstances that warrant a change in method. The same applies to antibody engineering, a field in which there are currently many alternative protocols. The book aims to provide enough information for the reader to decide which technique would be appropriate, to understand the power and major limitations of the techniques, and to find more information if necessary.

Glossary

This glossary concentrates on terms used in immunology to describe antibodies and the immune response leading to antibody production.

Affinity: A measure of the strength of binding between two molecular structures, for example antigenic epitope and the antigen binding site of antibody. Affinity is a precisely defined parameter, the ratio of the rate constants for association and dissociation (see also **avidity**).

Affinity chromatography: A family of techniques for purification of molecules based on their specific binding to other molecules on an inert solid support. Antibodies are frequently used to purify antigens from complex mixtures by coupling the antibody to a support, passing the mixture over this support so that everything except the specific antigen flows straight through, and then releasing (eluting) the bound antigen.

Affinity maturation: A process by which an early immune response, consisting of antibody which binds antigen weakly, is succeeded by the production of antibody which binds the antigen much more strongly. The basis of affinity maturation is the germinal center reaction, in which the immunoglobulin V region genes undergo a sequence of mutations and selection, such that mutations which increase affinity of the antibody for antigen are preserved, while cells carrying deleterious or null mutations are eliminated. Affinity maturation is strongly coupled to the generation of immunological memory, since a proportion of the selected, high-affinity antibody secreting cells are preserved as memory cells, ready to respond quickly and effectively if the same antigen is encountered again.

Avidity: Avidity measures the binding strength between antibody and antigen. Avidity differs from affinity in being a measure of the actual binding strength, as opposed to the strength of binding of individual binding sites. Avidity thus depends on affinity, but also on the number of binding sites (valency) and on other factors such as cooperativity of binding sites.

B cell precursors (progenitors): Cells early in differentiation which are committed to becoming B cells. B cell commitment takes the form of rearrangement of immunoglobulin genes, in preparation for immunoglobulin synthesis.

B lymphocyte: Cells responsible for antibody production.

C domain: Protein domains of antibody molecules which do not include the antigen-binding site, but are important in giving antibody its structural and biological properties.

CDR: See **V region**.

Cloning: In the context of hybridomas, cloning means isolating a single hybridoma cell and growing a population of identical cells from it. More generally cloning means isolating a single member of a population and producing multiple copies.

Complement: A term used to describe a series of proteins in serum, which have enzyme activities and are involved in the immune response. Typically, when antibody binds antigen, for example bacteria, it initiates a cascade of reactions involving a series of complement proteins and culminating in the destruction of the bacteria and the release of complement products that initiate further immunological reactions to ensure complete elimination of the foreign organism.

Conditioned medium: A term applied to the culture medium from a cell culture, usually after the cells have secreted something useful into the medium. Thus conditioned medium from a hybridoma would contain monoclonal antibody, while conditioned medium from a T cell culture might contain cytokines which help hybridoma cells to grow.

ELISA: Enzyme-linked immunoassay: A popular set of methods for measuring antibodies and antigens – there are many different forms of ELISA, and some of them are described in *Chapters 2, 4* and *5*.

Epitope: A molecular structure, part of an antigen, that directly interacts with antibody. Typically, a protein will contain multiple epitopes; i.e. antibodies can be made reacting with many different parts of the molecule.

Fab: Antibody fragment consisting of the entire light chain and the heavy chain V region with the first constant domain. See *Chapter 3* for detail.

Fc: Originally the crystallizable fragment of immunoglobulin, Fc is the portion involved in many of the biological functions of immunoglobulin, but not in antigen binding. See *Chapter 1* for detail.

Freund's complete adjuvant: The most widely used adjuvant in experimental animal immunization; stimulates strong, prolonged and high-affinity antibody responses.

Freund's incomplete adjuvant: Similar to Freund's complete adjuvant, but lacking the mycobacterial component. The mycobacteria boost responses, but should not be administered more than once to an animal, because of the risk of precipitating a fatal anaphylactic shock response. Therefore, the common approach is to use complete adjuvant for the priming injection and incomplete adjuvant for subsequent injections.

HAT medium: Selection medium to prevent unfused myeloma cells from growing and allow hybridomas to grow. The A (aminopterin) blocks the main biosynthetic pathway of DNA synthesis, while H and T (hypoxanthine and thymidine) fuel the salvage pathways. Myeloma lines used for fusion are defective in one or more enzymes of the salvage pathway and so cannot utilize HT; hybridomas have the necessary enzymes from the B cell fusion partner.

Hybridoma: The fusion product (hybrid) between a myeloma cell and a normal B cell, hybridomas are stable, rapidly dividing cell lines making monoclonal antibody.

IgA: Class of antibody, specialized for secretion onto mucosal surfaces.

IgG: The principal immunoglobulin class in the circulation and the major antibody against protein antigens. IgG is made by cells which initially made IgM but went through a class-switching to IgG; since this class switching process occurs in the germinal center reaction, also the site of affinity maturation, IgG are usually mutated and selected for high affinity.

IgM: Class of antibody, usually the first to be produced in response to a new antigenic challenge. IgM antibodies often have not been through the process of affinity maturation and lack mutations; the low affinity of the binding site is compensated for by the high valency (IgM is a pentamer of IgG-like divalent structures, so each IgM molecule has a potential valency of 10). IgM is the principal antibody class for antigens which do not engage T cell help, that is nonprotein antigens.

Memory B lymphocyte: Progeny of B cells which have been activated by antigen in conjunction with T lymphocyte signals; these cells usually make antibody of high affinity (see **affinity maturation**).

MHC: The major histocompatibility complex. The name refers to the complex of gene loci which determine tissue compatibility, i.e. tissues transplanted between individuals who differ in MHC antigens are rejected. The MHC proteins are now known to function in the interaction between T lymphocytes and antigen-presenting cells, an interaction which is central to immune responses to protein antigens.

Monoclonal antibody: A uniform population of antibody molecules (see also **polyclonal antibody**). All molecules in a monoclonal antibody population have the same binding specificity and affinity and the same biological properties – they should all have the same amino acid sequence, because they are produced by a population of identical cells (a single clone of cells, hence monoclonal).

Naive B lymphocyte: B cells which have not previously interacted with antigen.

Opsonization: Coating of particles (such as bacteria) with antibody and complement, which makes them susceptible to ingestion and killing by phagocytic cells of the immune system (macrophages and granulocytes).

PCR: Polymerase chain reaction: a family of techniques for making many copies of a particular DNA sequence, widely used analytically and in construction of molecular structures.

Phage display: A technique for expressing peptide or protein sequences (including antibody V regions) on the surface of filamentous phage. The gene coding the peptide is inserted into the phage genome, so that phage selected through the peptide's binding properties brings the appropriate gene with it. This coupling of gene to peptide makes phage display particularly useful as a method of affinity-selecting peptides from a large library.

Plasma cell: Terminally differentiated B cell, specialized for antibody secretion.

Polyclonal antibody: A preparation containing many different antibodies, even against the same antigen. Typically produced by immunizing an animal and isolating the immunoglobulin fraction from the serum.

Protein A: A bacterial protein which binds to some immunoglobulin isotypes and is therefore useful in the purification of antibodies.

Protein G: Like protein A, but protein G has a wider reactivity and can be used to purify all IgG antibodies.

scFv: Single-chain variable fragment: a minimal antibody molecule containing the heavy and light chain variable regions linked by a peptide chain. See *Chapter 3* for details.

Somatic mutation and selection: See **Affinity maturation.**

T lymphocyte: Immune cells responsible for 'cell mediated responses' such as transplant rejection and killing of virus-infected cells; T lymphocytes control B cell responses to protein antigens and T–B cell interaction is essential for the generation of high affinity antibody responses and memory B cells.

V region: The protein domain (or the DNA sequence coding for it) which includes the antigen-binding site. The heavy and light chains have one V region each (VH and VL). Each V region contains three hypervariable sequences flanked by framework sequences; the framework has a relatively rigid β-barrel structure while the hypervariable regions protrude as peptide loops. These loops are the primary sites of interaction with antigen and are called the complementarity-determining regions (CDR).

Valency: The number of binding sites per molecule.

The Basics

Chapter 1

Antibodies as laboratory and therapeutic reagents

H Zola

1. Introduction: antibody specificity and diversity

Antibodies are one of nature's answers to the need for a versatile system to recognize and dispose of foreign organisms or substances. The more complex species of animals are constantly challenged by viruses, bacteria and small parasites. Higher animals have evolved an immune system which allows an animal to rid itself of parasites, or at least to live in equilibrium with them. The diversity of potential pathogens, and their ability to evolve rapidly, has elicited an immune system which is capable of matching diversity and, uniquely, is able to evolve during the life of an individual.

The genes coding for antibody are assembled from a series of components in a manner which allows the permutation and combination of elements to produce an enormous diversity of sequences (estimated at 10^{11}). The antibody genes are then subjected to a process of somatic mutation which generates further diversity. This mutation is coupled with a mechanism for selection of the 'fittest' antibodies – those which bind foreign antigen that is present at the time. This combination of mutation and selection justifies the claim that the immune system is capable of evolving *during the life of an individual* to meet changing antigenic challenges. The results of this evolution are not generally thought to be passed to the germ cells and therefore are not thought to be inherited by the next generation. The mechanisms of mutation and selection occurring within the cells responsible for antibody production (B lymphocytes) allow antibody to evolve to meet immunological challenges, within the lifetime of the individual and indeed within days.

With an emerging understanding of the function of antibody it did not take immunologists long to realize that this natural defense mechanism could be put to use in the laboratory or in the treatment of disease. The ability to generate molecules capable of highly specific molecular recognition, and to apply this approach to virtually any molecular target, makes antibody technology powerful. It may be instructive to compare antibodies with enzymes. Enzymes are highly specific catalysts of biochemical reactions. There are a large number of enzymes, but the number is nevertheless limited. If the reaction you wish to catalyze does not occur anywhere in nature, you won't find an enzyme to catalyze it. You may be able to design one, and construct it, but the enzyme system is not designed for infinite versatility, as the antibody system is. Indeed, biologists who want to design novel catalysts are now basing them on antibody structures.

2. Antibody specificity: protein structure

How specific are antibodies? We know from experience or observation that an attack of measles protects us from a subsequent attack of measles, but not from German measles. The immune system distinguishes the two viruses. An attack of influenza will protect us from subsequent attacks for a short time, but the virus is constantly mutating and next year we may well encounter a related but somewhat different virus, and our immunological memory of the previous exposure will not prevent illness (though it does greatly reduce the severity of the disease).

We can examine specificity at a molecular level. The blood group antibodies which determine which types of blood can be transfused safely into an individual distinguish glycoproteins which differ by only one sugar. Monoclonal antibodies made against glycoproteins can distinguish structures which differ only in the modification of a sugar residue – acetylation of an amino group, for example.

How is this specificity determined? The structure of the antibody molecule is illustrated schematically in *Figures 1.1* and *1.2*, while *Figure 1.3* shows the structure of a typical antibody binding site for antigen. Constant domains consist of beta barrels formed from seven beta-strands (*Figure 1.2*). Variable domains have a similar structure, but have three protruding polypeptide loops. One of the beta-barrels, with its three loops, forms the V (variable) domain of the immunoglobulin heavy chain, while another beta-barrel with its three loops forms the V domain of the light chain. The binding site consists principally of the six peptide loops, the complementarity-determining regions (CDR).

While the beta-barrel structure is relatively invariant in sequence and structure between different antibodies, the CDR loops are highly variable in sequence and hence in their ability to interact with antigen.

The binding of antigen by antibody consists of interactions between the CDR loops and the antigen (*Figure 1.3*). These interactions may be

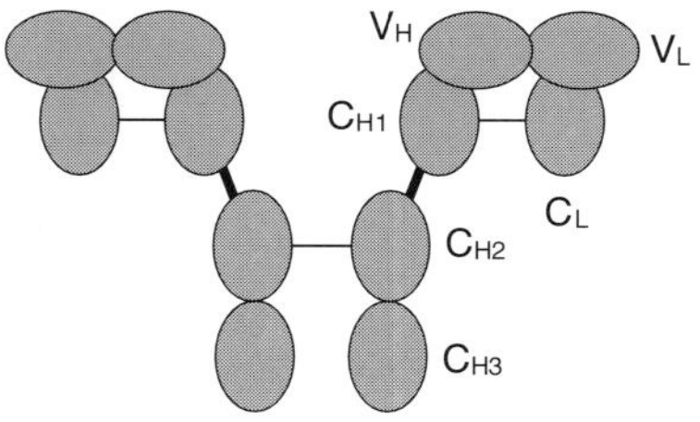

Figure 1.1

Antibody structures: Arrangement of the constant (C) and variable (V) region domains (each domain is shown as an oval and the standard abbreviations are shown). Thin lines linking domains represent disulfide bonds, while the thick lines linking C_{H1} to C_{H2} is the flexible part of the amino acid sequence called the hinge region.

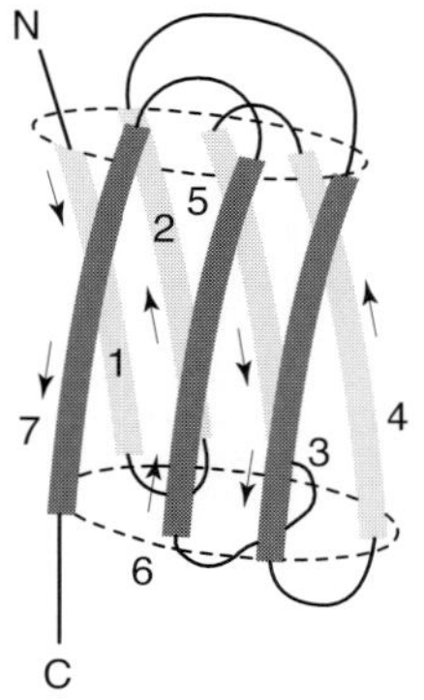

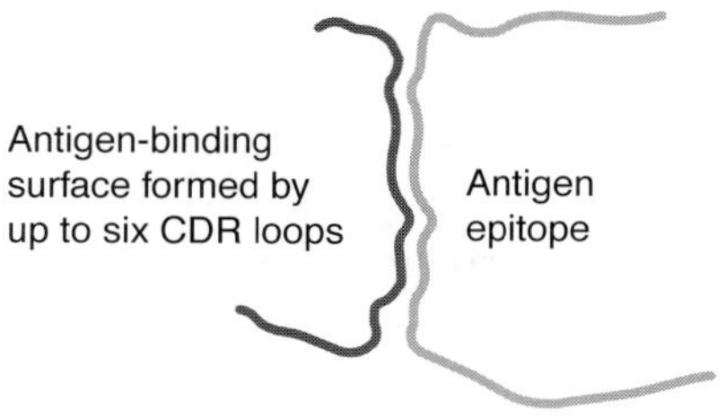

Figure 1.3

Representation of the antigen-binding surface of Ig.

Figure 1.2

Arrangement of seven beta strands into a beta barrel in the typical immunoglobulin constant domain. The strands are numbered in sequence from the N terminus, and arrows follow the N–C direction.

hydrophobic interactions, charge interactions or a mixture of both. The binding may involve all six CDRs or fewer, and the area of interaction is the major determinant of the affinity, which is a measure of strength of binding. A change in one amino acid residue may change binding affinity significantly. Mutations outside the CDR can have a dramatic effect on binding of antigen, because the beta strands that form the barrel structure provide the framework on which the CDR loops are built, and a change in framework can completely alter the orientation of the loop.

3. The immunoglobulin constant region: form and functions

The antibody molecule (see *Figure 1.1*) has an antigen-binding site, which has been described in detail in the previous section. This antigen-binding site consists of the variable domains of the light and heavy chains, V_L and V_H, linked to constant domains C_L and C_{H1}. The rest of the molecule (called the Fc portion) consists of the C_{H2} and C_{H3} domains (*Figure 1.2*) and mediates most of the functions of antibody. Once antibody has bound a pathogen, for example a bacterial cell, other mechanisms must be brought into play to remove it – mechanisms such as the uptake of antibody-coated bacteria by macrophages – these are mediated by the Fc.

The antibody molecule and the cells of the immune system have evolved together to provide a variety of immunological mechanisms. Macrophages, neutrophils and several other cell types have receptors for the Fc part of immunoglobulin which facilitate the removal of antibody coated antigen. Variety in immune mechanisms is conferred by having multiple forms of the Fc and multiple receptors expressed by different cell types. Thus IgA is the immunoglobulin characteristic of mucosal secretions, and cells of the mucosal immune system have IgA receptors (Fc-alpha receptors); IgE is particularly effective in combating some of the larger parasites, with the help of mast cells which have specific receptors for IgE.

The Ig isoforms are shown in *Figures 1.4–1.6*, and their major properties are tabulated in *Table 1.1*. The genes coding for these Fc isoforms are arranged, downstream from the V region genes, in the sequence: μ, δ, $\gamma3$, $\gamma1$, $\alpha1$, $\gamma2$, ε, and $\alpha2$, where the Greek letter is used to denote the heavy chain (δ for IgD, etc) . IgM is generally the first isoform secreted, followed by IgG

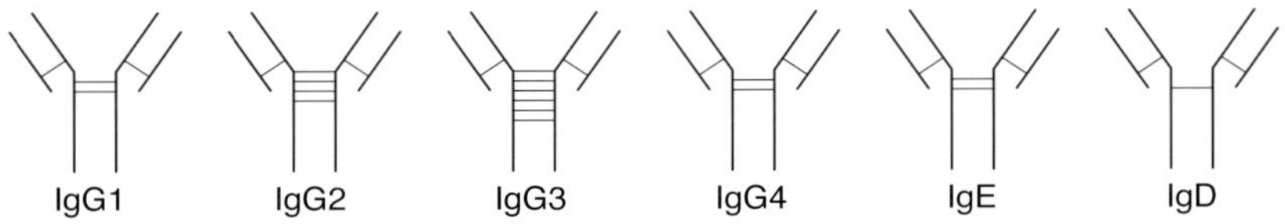

Figure 1.4

The IgG subclasses, IgE and IgD in humans. IgD is principally a cell-surface Ig. IgE has an extra CH domain, giving it a higher molecular weight. Mice have analogous IgG isotypes, referred to as IgG1, 2a, 2b, and 3.

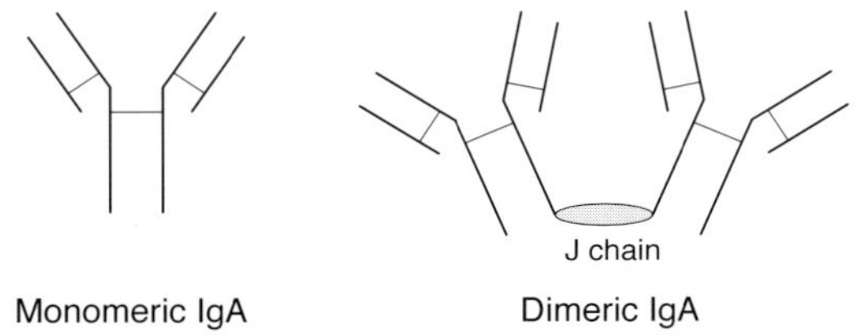

Figure 1.5

Monomeric and dimeric IgA. IgA in secretions is largely in the dimeric form associated with J chain, and is additionally associated with a protein called secretory piece.

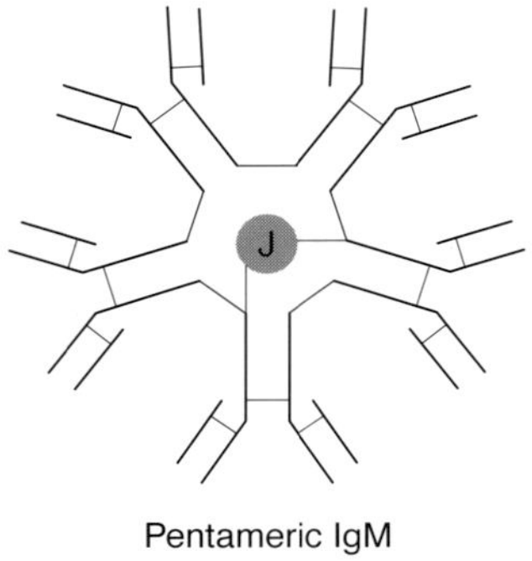

Figure 1.6

The standard, pentameric form of IgM.

variants (IgD is largely restricted to the cell membrane) and IgA or IgE are secreted only in special circumstances or tissues.

For the practical purposes of the antibody maker, IgE and IgA are rarely encountered among monoclonals. IgM antibodies result from a primary response, or in response to nonprotein antigens (see below). IgM are generally more difficult to work with than IgG. Even among the four subclasses of IgG there are significant differences in binding to Fc receptors and therefore in function and in non-specific staining of cells and tissue.

Table 1.1 Properties of the mouse Ig isoforms most commonly produced by hybridomas.

Property	IgG1	IgG2a	IgG2b	IgG3	IgM
Heavy chain	γ1	γ2a	γ2b	γ3	μ
Valency	2	2	2	2	up to 10
Complement fixing	–	+	+++	+	+++
Major features	Common hybridoma product	Common hybridoma product	Rare hybridoma product	Often carbohydrate antigens	Early response, carbohydrate antigens
Protein A binding[a]	pH>8	pH>4.5	pH>3.5	pH>4.5	–
Protein G binding[a]	+	+	+	+	+/–

[a]Protein A and Protein G are bacterial proteins that bind some immunoglobulin isotypes and are useful for the purification of these antibody types.

4. The cells that make antibody

Antibodies are made by B lymphocytes. B cells originate from common hematopoietic progenitors which give rise to all the blood cells, and differentiate through a number of stages, to the terminally differentiated plasma cell, which produces soluble antibody. As hematopoietic stem cells differentiate the first cell that can be recognized as a B cell precursor is a cell that has begun to rearrange its immunoglobulin genes, in the manner described in the next section. A succession of B cell precursor stages can be recognized, with increasingly modified immunoglobulin gene sequences, until the cell is able to express immunoglobulin as a cell membrane protein. Cells expressing antibody on the surface are called B cells, the entire cycle including precursors and later differentiated forms are collectively referred to as belonging to the B cell lineage. B cells go through a defined series of differentiation stages, during which they express the different immunoglobulin isotypes, they undergo proliferation if they encounter antigen, they may enter the process of somatic mutation and selection described in the next section, and they may eventually differentiate into either memory cells or plasma cells. The life cycle of B cells is summarized in *Figure 1.7*.

Memory B cells have been specifically activated in interaction with antigen and the T cell component of the immune system. They differ from naive (previously unstimulated) B cells in that they are poised to respond to a later exposure to the same antigen in a vigorous and highly effective manner, proliferating rapidly to give rise to plasma cells that make antibody that binds the antigen with high affinity. These antibodies are usually of the IgG, IgA, or IgE isotypes and are in some ways more effective than the IgM antibodies characteristic of a primary antibody response. *Figure 1.8* summarizes the differences between a primary and a secondary response.

Plasma cells are specialized antibody factories, with a highly-developed endoplasmic reticulum dedicated to assembling and secreting antibody. While the immunoglobulin of B cells has a hydrophobic sequence which keeps it anchored in the cell membrane, plasma cells make a shortened immunoglobulin molecule which is secreted.

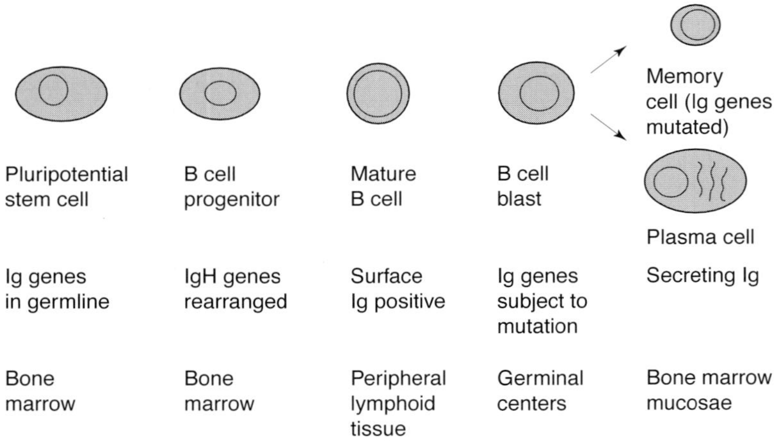

Figure 1.7

B cell differentiation: The principal stages of B cell differentiation, with principal defining characteristics and major locations.

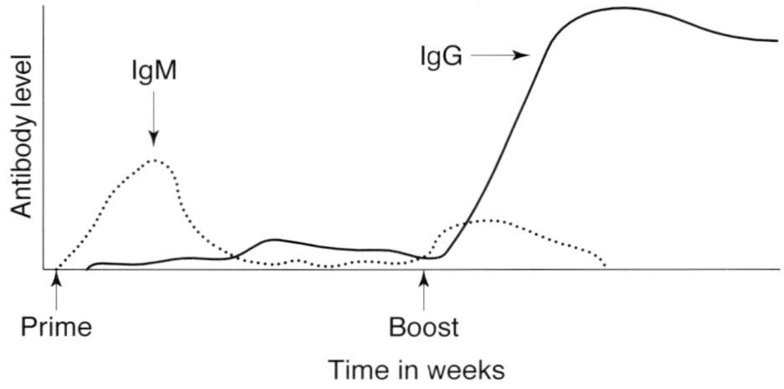

Figure 1.8

Primary and secondary responses.

5. The basis of antibody specificity and diversity: unique genetic mechanisms

The genes coding the antibody variable domain are assembled from a set of genetic elements. A heavy chain V region is assembled from three elements – V (variable), D (diversity) and J (joining). The light chain is simpler, consisting of only V and J elements. The region that codes for the heavy chain contains approximately 50 usable V elements, about 10 D elements and 4 J sequences. There are additional V genes which are not used, which explains why you will find the number of alternative V regions described as anywhere between 50 and 1000 depending on which textbook you use. The light chains are coded somewhat differently but the general principle – combination of a V and a J selected from a menu of available sequences – is the same.

When a B cell precursor matures into a B cell, a random permutation of VDJ and VJ elements occurs. The diversity available by permutation between 50 V, 10 D, and 4 J elements is 2000; this is increased because any heavy chain combination can in principle be paired with any light chain combination, but the diversity is greatly increased by another factor. When any two elements (V and D, or an assembled VD and J) are brought together and joined, the joining is imprecise – nucleotides may be added or subtracted. This greatly increases the overall number of antibody sequences, to an estimated 10^{11}, and is the major mechanism allowing higher animals to respond immunologically to new mutants of pathogens. One indication of the magnitude of this diversity achieved by manipulation of a small number of genetic elements is that the total number of genes required to code for an entire higher animal is about 10^5.

This is not the limit of the versatility of the antibody system, however. The final antibody binding site sequence and hence structure is, for many antibody molecules, reached in two stages. The first is Ig gene rearrangements as just described. This process is random and continues all the time, whatever the antigenic challenges prevalent at the time. By chance an invading organism will be detected by a B lymphocyte bearing on its surface an antibody which binds one of the many molecules on the surface of the pathogen (and the number 10^{11} makes such a chance encounter probable). This initial interaction between the pathogen and the immune system can lead to a cascade of reactions which induce proliferation of the cell making the antibody, involvement of other components of the immune system, a spreading of the antibody response so that multiple antibodies are made against multiple antigens of the pathogen, and finally a process called affinity maturation, which results in an increase in the average binding affinity of the antibodies for the molecules of the pathogen. Affinity maturation is the second stage determining the binding site structure. It results in a fine-tuning rather than a wholesale redesigning of the binding site. Typically, it results in an increase in the contact area between antigen and antibody. The CDR3 is the major site of variation resulting from the process of gene rearrangement (because it contains the VDJ or VJ junctions, including junctional insertions and deletions); mutations often affect CDR1 and 2 as well as CDR3.

The process of affinity maturation involves mutation of the immunoglobulin genes coupled to selection of B cells bearing antibody of the highest affinity. This process has much in common with Darwinian evolution. The mutations are random. This statement requires qualification. The mutational machinery is selective in that it targets only the variable region sequences, and some types of mutations are more likely than others. These features reflect aspects of the mutational machinery, but the process of mutation is random in that it does not selectively produce mutations which lead to higher affinity. Indeed, since it is much easier to damage a binding site than to improve the area of contact, it is likely that the vast majority of mutations are deleterious to binding affinity. The improvement of affinity is due to the coupling of mutation to a process of selection, just as it is in Darwinian selection on the basis of fitness. Fitness in Darwinian evolution means the ability for the gene to propagate itself by conferring on the whole organism an advantage in reproductive success rate. In the case of antibody genes it is the B cells that derive an advantage in reproductive capacity from an improved antigen-binding affinity. The tissue site of affinity maturation (the germinal center) contains specialized cells (follicular dendritic cells) which retain antigen, and T cells which react with B cells that have internalized antigen. B cells proliferate and in the process mutate their antibody genes. The B cell progeny are induced to die (apoptosis) unless they receive strong survival signals both from follicular dendritic cells and from T cells.

The net result is a rapid multiplication of B cells accompanied by diversification of the antigen-binding site, followed by death of the majority and retention only of those with increased binding affinity. The diversification reinforces the homology with Darwinian evolution, which leads to diversification of species, not just increased fitness of a single species.

When antibody genes are sequenced the effects of mutation and selection leave characteristic footprints. Mutation without selection results in an essentially random distribution of replacement mutations in the CDR and framework regions of the antibody V domain, while mutation coupled with selection leads to clustering of replacement mutations in the CDR. Framework mutations are selected against because they have a high probability of destabilizing the binding site. Silent mutations (mutations which change a codon to a different codon that specifies the same amino acid) are randomly distributed whether or not selection is operating.

Significantly for antibody technology, mutation and selection operate for protein antigens but not for nonprotein antigens, such as carbohydrates and lipids. Some affinity maturation can be seen with these antigens, but it is different in mechanism and in effectiveness. As the amount of antigen available becomes limiting late in an immune response, only those B cells with high affinity for antigen are likely to bind antigen and be stimulated. Affinity maturation in this situation operates by selecting among immunoglobulin gene rearrangements, without mutation.

The practical result of the way carbohydrate and lipid antigens are handled by the immune system is that antibodies against these antigens are often of relatively low affinity. They tend also to be IgM, because the process of class switching from IgM to IgG is also located in the germinal center, although it operates independently from mutation and selection. As will be seen later, IgM antibodies are generally less easy to work with than IgG.

6. Polyclonal antisera

Let us now examine the antibody response as seen at the level of the whole animal. We immunize say a rabbit and the processes discussed in the previous section occur. We bleed the rabbit after 2–4 weeks and examine the serum for antibodies. The serum will contain the products of many germinal centers, many B cells making a variety of antibodies against each antigenic structure on the injected antigen (the immunogen). If the immunogen was a viral or bacterial suspension there may be hundreds of different antibodies. If the immunogen was a pure protein there will still be probably tens of different antibodies. Furthermore, the serum will contain additional antibodies against antigens previously encountered by the rabbit. Indeed, if we find that 1% of the immunoglobulin in the serum is directed against our immunogen of interest we will consider we have done very well. To take a specific example, if we sample the blood of a human subject who has recently been boosted with the tetanus toxoid antigen the B cells which can specifically recognize tetanus toxoid comprise approximately 0.3% of the B cells in the sample. We can expect the proportion of antibody reacting with tetanus toxoid to be of the same order.

Thus in spite of the specificity of individual antibodies and individual B cells, the serum is a rich mixture of many different antibodies, against the same antigen and against many different antigens. Notwithstanding the rich mixture, antibodies were powerful reagents for laboratory and clinical use before the advent of monoclonal antibodies. Antisera were used for anything from pregnancy testing to the treatment of gas gangrene or snake-bite envenomation, and were considered a major advance on methods that preceded them. Take pregnancy testing, or any other hormone assay that can be done with confidence using an antibody. These immunoassays replaced bioassays, where the pregnancy hormones were detected by injecting a urine sample into a small animal and looking for the physiological consequences. The animal-based assay for insulin, which involved inducing a diabetic coma in rats, was a particularly unpleasant assay, with limited precision. Immunoassays were a great improvement both in sparing a large number of animals (a small number of rabbits will make enough antiserum for a large number of immunoassays) and in increasing assay speed and precision. It was always necessary to remember the reagent was a mixture, and to look out for spurious results due to the presence of a contaminating antibody.

7. Monoclonal antibodies

The aim of the monoclonal antibody approach to making antibodies is to take advantage of the fact that a single B cell makes only one antibody specificity – one set of six CDRs, whether mutated or not. The strategy is to clone the B cells from an immunized animal.

The original method, described by Kohler and Milstein in 1975, is to take the lymphocytes from the spleen of an immunized mouse and make hybridomas, fusion products between the mouse B lymphocytes and myeloma cells. Myelomas are malignant antibody-secreting cells, and the myeloma lines used proliferate rapidly and secrete large amounts of antibodies. Large numbers of fusion products can result from the fusion of myeloma and B cells; these cells initially contain the full complement of genes from both parent cells, but then randomly lose some of the genes. Among the fusion products will be cells which proliferate rapidly and secrete large amounts of antibody, coded for by the genes from the spleen cells.

Even amongst these cells, the hybridomas secreting antibody against the antigen of interest will be a minority (see the discussion above on the proportion of cells reactive with a particular antigen). However, the hybridomas can be cloned, that is, placed in small culture vessels such that each culture contains initially a single cell, and later the identical progeny of that cell. If we have an assay to screen large numbers of cultures for antibody reactive against the antigen of interest, we have the basis for the production of monoclonal antibodies at will against antigens of our choosing.

8. The major differences between monoclonal and polyclonal antibodies

A solution of monoclonal antibody consists of identical molecules, with identical specificity, affinity for antigen, and ability to engage biological processes such as opsonization (the coating of bacteria with antibody and serum proteins collectively called complement, to make them ingestible by phagocytic cells). A solution of antibody derived from serum, in contrast, contains a mixture of antibodies. There will be antibodies against unrelated antigens, antibodies against several epitopes of the antigen of interest; even among antibodies against the same epitope there will be antibodies of differing affinity, and there will be antibodies of differing subclass and consequently different biological properties.

There is a mixture of antibodies within a polyclonal sample; there is also variety between samples. Here the difference between polyclonal and monoclonal samples is not as great as it might seem. A large bleed from a rabbit or larger animal can be divided into many small aliquots and stored, we can return to identical samples time after time for several years. Different bleeds from the same rabbit may differ significantly in composition and activity. Monoclonal antibodies have the theoretical advantage that, once you have isolated a stable clone, you can produce identical antibody indefinitely for years. In practice, it is still necessary to check this, to perform quality control. Cultures harvested at different times are unlikely to vary qualitatively, but the amount of antibody secreted can vary considerably. Furthermore, storage and handling can affect antibody function, whether monoclonal or polyclonal. In particular a sample that has been frozen and thawed may lose some activity and may contain aggregates which contribute to nonspecific binding. This can happen with monoclonal or polyclonal antibodies equally.

Polyclonality is not all bad. A polyclonal sample will contain multiple antibodies against different parts of the antigen molecule or particle, and this greatly enhances reactivity in most types of assay. Reactions such as precipitation of antigen by antibody (immunoprecipitation) depend on cross-linking of antigen and antibody in a large aggregate which becomes insoluble. If the antigen has multiple copies of an epitope per molecule (for example a polysaccharide), a monoclonal antibody against the epitope can form large aggregates and cause precipitation. However, if the epitope is present only once per molecule (typical for a protein antigen), the best a bivalent antibody can achieve is a string of molecules linked together, which may or may not precipitate (*Figure 1.9a*). In this situation a polyclonal serum would probably contain antibodies against several different epitopes on the molecule, and would therefore achieve cross-linking and precipitation (*Figure 1.9b*). Even in reactions such as agglutination of cells, where multiple

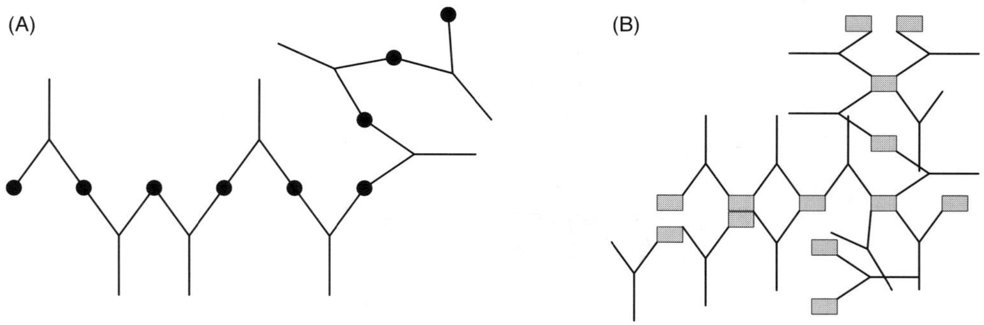

Figure 1.9

Diagram showing cross-linking and aggregate formation. (A) Interaction between a bivalent antibody and bivalent antigen can only produce 'strings' of antigen–antibody, which generally do not precipitate. (B) Larger, precipitating aggregates are produced if either the antibody or the antigen has a valency greater than two.

copies of each epitope are available, polyclonal antibodies generally give a stronger reaction, because of the presence of antibodies against several different epitopes. The same applies to reactions such as immunofluorescence, where cross-linking is not necessary, simply because of the presence of multiple antibodies in polyclonal sera.

As a general rule a polyclonal antiserum will give a stronger signal than a monoclonal antibody in any immunological test procedure. This stronger signal must be balanced against the greater risk of a confounding cross-reaction in the polyclonal preparation, and the greater control of batch–batch reproducibility with monoclonal antibodies. The balance comes out in favour of monoclonal antibodies in some applications, polyclonal antibodies in others. There are fields of application where monoclonal antibodies have almost completely replaced polyclonals, and have greatly extended the analytical power of immunoassay, by uncovering an antigenic complexity which was beyond the analytical power of polyclonal sera. An example is the analysis of the cell surface molecules of leukocytes (see *Chapter 6*). The complexity of these cell surface molecules (currently represented by 168 'CD' molecules) was not even dreamed about in the early 1970s, when polyclonal sera identified T and B cells, and showed that T cells were not all the same. On the other hand, immunoassays for a variety of hormones are still carried out with polyclonal antisera, and there is no pressing reason to change. The assays work well, and there is no known risk of cross-reactivity.

When working in a new field, where the complexity of the molecules being studied, and therefore the risk of cross-reactivity, are not known, it is safer to work with monoclonal antibodies if possible. This is to reduce the risk of reaching conclusions which turn out, later, to be confounded by the presence of a second, related molecule, or a cross-reaction with an unrelated molecule. Since the preparation of monoclonal antibodies is more complex, time-consuming and unpredictable than the preparation of a polyclonal antiserum, a reasonable approach with a new molecule is to make a polyclonal antiserum first, and follow that up with a monoclonal antibody, always remembering that the results obtained with polyclonal antisera are at risk of being confounded by cross-reactions.

9. Applications of antibodies in the laboratory

Antibodies have achieved widespread use in laboratories working on all aspects of medicine and biology. Antibodies are well suited to any situation where molecular recognition can be used to identify, quantify, localize or purify a molecule or cell (*Figure 1.10*). This section illustrates the power of antibody-based laboratory techniques by giving specific examples; methodology is covered in later Chapters.

9.1 Identification

The specificity of the antigen–antibody reaction, coupled with inherent biological variation, makes antibody a highly specific reagent for identifying individual molecules in complex mixtures, and distinguishing related molecules. Antibody-based reactions are used to identify genetic variants of blood cells to avoid transfusion of inappropriate blood type and to reduce the severity of transplant rejection. Antibodies can be used to identify the species of origin of blood or tissue in forensic applications, and the infecting pathogen in the diagnosis of infection.

9.2 Localization

If the antibody can identify a molecule it is a logical extension to use the antibody, together with a suitable staining reaction and a microscope, to localize molecules in tissue. Immunohistology, as the technique is called,

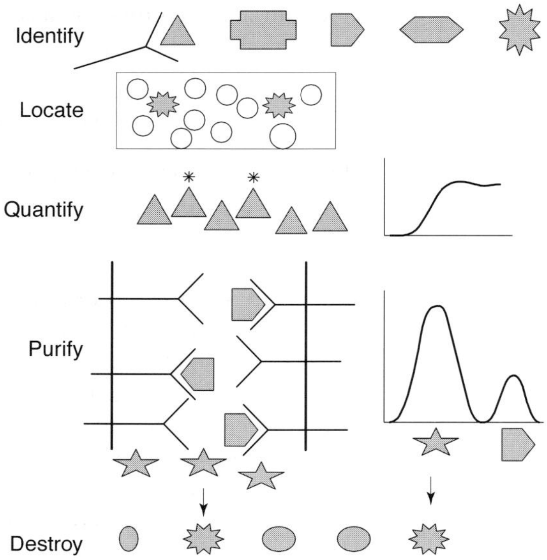

Figure 1.10

Schematic representation of antibody applications.

has proved powerful in the diagnosis of disease, localizing pathogens, malignant cells, or components of the immune system in infected, malignant or inflamed tissue.

9.3 Quantitation

The finding of IgE in the serum means nothing to the pathologist investigating the cause of a set of symptoms in a patient. But the finding that IgE levels are much higher than in the general population suggests an allergic disease, and indicates some more specific tests that will be more informative, possibly confirming allergy and identifying the major allergen. The presence of thyroid hormone in serum is again of little significance, but the presence of a greatly reduced level of hormone suggests a diagnosis and treatment. In many situations in medicine and biology what is important is not so much the presence of a particular molecule, but the quantity present. Where an antibody can identify a molecule, a change in assay format can provide quantitative information.

A molecule can serve as a marker for a particular type of cell – the CD4 molecule for the cells that are the primary target of the AIDS virus, for example. The number of cells can then be counted. This is different from quantitation of the molecule itself, and provides another dimension to antibody-based quantitative analysis.

9.4 Purification

The methods discussed in the preceding paragraphs are analytical, but antibodies also provide powerful reagents for preparative applications. Antibodies can be used to purify molecules by affinity chromatography, or to purify cells bearing markers detected by the antibody. Affinity-based purification methods are often much more powerful than conventional biochemical procedures, because they can distinguish molecules having generally similar properties.

10. Therapeutic applications of antibodies

The use of antibody for therapy has a long history, going back at least to 1890 and the use by von Behring and Kitasato of antibodies made in horses to neutralize diphtheria toxin. Although immunization has greatly reduced the incidence of infections such as tetanus, diphtheria, and gangrene, antisera are still used to reverse toxicity due to bacterial toxins and to the venoms of snakes, spiders and other venomous animals. Antibodies are highly effective in this situation, where what is required is a rapid reduction in the amount of toxin in the system, to allow time for other forms of treatment and the patient's own immune system to provide a cure. A major problem associated with the use of antibodies, the development of an immune response against the injected antibody (itself a foreign protein), is less likely to be important in this situation as few people get bitten by snakes twice.

The use of antibodies to neutralize foreign toxins provides but one type of application. A conceptually distinct use of antibodies is to rid the body of abnormal self-constituents such as cancer cells, and another, conceptually distinct again, is to control the level of normal self molecules, cells or processes, for example to dampen down the immune system to allow a transplant of foreign tissue to establish itself.

The preparation of antibodies for cancer therapy has a checkered history. Initial optimism was tempered by a lack of success, and by a realization that belief in the widespread existence of tumor specific target antigens was the product of wishful thinking rather than solid evidence. A sober re-examination of the antigenicity of tumors allowed two positive factors to survive. The first is that the genetic translocations that we now know to underlie many malignancies can code for new proteins, and these proteins may be antigenic. They are not necessarily expressed on the surface at a level that would allow antibody-mediated killing, but they are in some tumors. Furthermore, they are likely to be expressed as peptide fragments in association with the membrane protein major histocompatibility complex (MHC) Class I, thus serving as a potential target for T cell-mediated killing. The second encouraging factor is the realization that lineage-specific antigens, shared by the malignant cell and its normal counterpart, may be targeted, provided the normal counterpart cell is either not essential for survival or readily regenerated from precursors.

As a consequence of these concepts, and of the technical innovations to be described in the next section, immunotherapy of cancer is undergoing a renaissance. There have been spectacular successes in treatment of tumors with antibodies over the last decade, but they have been isolated. There is currently a new generation of monoclonal antibodies undergoing clinical trials, with promising results, and several have been approved for clinical use in the last few years.

The use of antibodies to control physiological process such as inflammation and the immune response itself is also the subject of much current activity and optimism. In the 1960s and 70s antilymphocyte sera were made in horses or smaller animals to use in reversing the transplant rejection reaction, which is mediated by lymphocytes. These polyclonal antisera were successful, but were largely replaced a few years later by a monoclonal antibody, OKT3. This antibody is directed against a component of the T cell receptor and incapacitates T cells. It was preferred over polyclonal antisera largely because its effects were reproducible and relatively predictable, and provides a prime example of the advantages of monoclonal over polyclonal antibodies.

For about 20 years OKT3 has been the only consistent example of therapeutic applications of monoclonal antibodies. Its unique success has served to emphasize the unfulfilled promise of monoclonal antibodies as therapeutic substances, in contrast to their many successes in the laboratory. Other antibodies have been trialed, either to improve on OKT3 or to treat acute inflammatory conditions, such as toxic shock syndrome, or chronic autoimmune conditions, such as rheumatoid arthritis. Several have shown promise, but until recently none have achieved widespread use. New reagents emerging from clinical trials seem set to change this picture.

The widespread use of OKT3 shows that, given appropriate therapeutic effectiveness, monoclonal antibodies will be used. However, there are a number of disadvantages to the use of whole antibodies derived from a different species. These will be discussed in detail in *Chapter 3*, but probably the most intractable one is the immunogenicity of these antibodies. As foreign proteins, they elicit an immune response in the patient. At best, this leads to their rapid clearance on subsequent exposure, at worst it can lead to a severe anaphylactic response on second or subsequent exposure.

Several of the limitations of monoclonal antibodies in therapeutic application can be overcome, at least in principle, by tailoring the antibody molecule to remove some segments and add others – antibody engineering.

11. Improving on nature – antibody engineering

The antibody molecule is a complex structure, with an antigen-binding segment and a larger segment which does not contribute to antigen binding, but determines the functional properties of the antibody. This evolved design of antibody has clearly suited its natural functions well, but different designs may suit our artificial applications of antibodies better. Antibodies have long been modified for use, in particular antibody used to neutralize toxins is often treated with protease to remove the Fc end, leaving bivalent antigen-binding fragments $F(ab)_2$, which consists of two $(V_H\text{-}C_{H1})\text{-}(V_L\text{-}C_L)$ structures linked by disulfide bonds (see *Figure 1.1*). Molecular biological techniques allow the modification of the antibody genes, as opposed to direct modification of the proteins. This has the major advantage that it has to be done once only; the modified genes can then be expressed, producing the modified antibody protein. The starting point for antibody engineering is normally the DNA from a hybridoma. Antibody engineering will be discussed in *Chapter 3*.

12. Replacing nature – antibodies from gene libraries

Suitable hybridomas are not always available to serve as a starting point for antibody engineering, and not all molecules are immunogenic. An approach which completely bypasses the need for animal immunization or hybridoma is to make a synthetic library of immunoglobulin V region genes, and to select from the library genes coding for structures that bind the antigen. The most widely used method to achieve this is the phage display method. The antibody genes are incorporated into bacteriophage, linked to a phage coat protein. When the phage are assembled, the antibody protein is expressed on the phage coat. Reaction with the antigen allows binding of phage coding for antibody with affinity for the antigen; the genes are coabsorbed with the antibody protein, as part of the phage. Once the phage has been cloned a change in conditions allows the protein to be produced as a soluble protein. Phage display and antibody libraries will be described in *Chapter 3*.

13. Conclusions

Antibodies have evolved as a powerful weapon against infection. Their specificity makes them powerful tools in the laboratory and as therapeutic agents. That specificity often cannot be realized fully by immunizing an animal and taking its serum; the monoclonal antibody technique allows full realization of the laboratory applications of antibody specificity. Therapeutic applications have been limited by some of the properties of the antibody molecule; it appears probable that antibody engineering will resolve many of these problems and therapeutic applications of antibodies are developing rapidly.

Further reading

The original paper describing the hybridoma technique:

Kohler, G. and Milstein, C. (1975) Continuous cultures of fused cells secreting antibody of predefined specificity. *Nature* **256**, 495–497.

Basic immunology texts for anyone wanting a better understanding of the immune system:

Roitt, I. (1997) *Essential Immunology,* 9th edn. Blackwell, Oxford.
Janeway, C.A. and Travers, P. *Immunobiology,* 4th edn. Current Biology, London.

The Basics

Chapter 2

Hybridoma technology: making monoclonal antibodies

B Hunt, H Zola and C Goddard

1. Introduction

The production of murine monoclonal antibodies is now a well established method, originally pioneered by Kohler and Milstein (1975). Many laboratories have subsequently developed the facilities and expertise for monoclonal antibody production although there are considerable differences between laboratories in methodology, and also a perceived element of 'black magic'. This chapter describes the 'conventional' technique for the production of monoclonal antibodies based on personal experiences of different protocols in several laboratories. It is not intended as an exhaustive review of all the methodology but attempts to provide the reader with an understanding of the technique and equipment required to develop monoclonal antibodies by established methods. The major requirements are an understanding of the theoretical basis behind the method, and sound cell culture technique.

2. Theoretical basis

A monoclonal antibody is produced by an immortal cell line derived from the fusion of a malignant myeloma cell with a B lymphocyte, usually derived from the spleen of an immunized mouse. The myeloma line is deficient in one of the essential salvage pathways for DNA synthesis and so does not survive when the main biosynthetic pathway for DNA synthesis is blocked. The unfused spleen derived lymphocytes do not survive because they are physiologically programmed to die unless 'rescued'. The only cells which survive in the appropriate medium are hybridomas, the myeloma-spleen cell hybrids resulting from the fusion. The hybridoma derives its immortality and antibody secreting capacity from the myeloma cell genes, and the salvage pathway genes and antibody-coding genes from the spleen B lymphocyte

3. Cell culture

3.1 Basic requirements

The basic requirements have changed little in the last few years apart from a general simplification of the procedure and standardization of critical reagents, which are now available commercially pretested for hybridoma use. The investment of time and resources can be considerable and there is no guarantee that a monoclonal antibody can be generated against a given molecule. Monoclonal antibodies have been generated against a very wide range of molecules and many are commercially available. Some companies offer to generate monoclonal antibodies against customer supplied antigen for a fee. About two months are required to immunize the mice, and a further three months to generate the hybridomas, screen for positive hybridomas, clone and cryopreserve.

Making monoclonal antibodies requires experience in cell culture and availability of some basic equipment, including a tissue culture laboratory and an animal house. The laboratory should have a sterile hood, a 37 °C 5% CO_2 gassed incubator, a centrifuge, an inverted microscope, water purification unit and liquid nitrogen storage facilities. Access to autoclave facilities is desirable, but the need to sterilize glassware is now generally overcome by purchasing sterile disposable plasticware. If all of these (particularly tissue culture experience) are available, the preparation of hybridomas can be undertaken with confidence. If they are not available, it will probably be better to pay for a contract researcher to make them, or seek a collaborator with the necessary experience and facilities.

In any cell culture laboratory things go wrong from time to time; cells stop growing, infections occur and reagents lose activity. Most of these problems can be overcome by appropriate Good Laboratory Practice. Sterile technique is essential in tissue culture laboratories; production of monoclonal antibodies requires months of tissue culture. For a good text on general tissue culture methodology, see Freshney (1983). The major consumable costs include tissue culture flasks and microtiter plates, media and fetal bovine serum (FBS). An outlay in the order of US$1000 (1999) is required on consumables. Ethics approval must be obtained from the relevant authority before immunization can begin.

The sequence of events in making monoclonal antibodies is shown in *Table 2.1*. After the last step you should be in a position to grow up quantities of monoclonal antibody for use. At each point we emphasize cryopreservation, as the only insurance against loss of useful cultures.

3.2 Materials

All the materials needed to produce monoclonal antibodies can be purchased. The quality of cell culture reagents from most commercial sources is good, and we have not specified particular brands except where we believe there is significant variation.

Cell culture medium

The two culture media used in most laboratories are Dulbecco's minimum essential medium (DMEM) and RPMI 1640. We have not experienced major differences in performance between them and both are available in liquid or powder form. The powder form must be sterilized once dissolved. The quality of water is critical. We use water from a well maintained water purification unit although commercially available 'water-for-injection' is an alternative. Note that water purification units for different purposes produce

Table 2.1. Schedule for making monoclonal antibodies.

1.	Prepare antigen and develop screening assay.
2.	Immunize animals, a minimum of two for each antigen.
3.	One week before fusion, thaw myeloma cells and scale-up. About 10^8 cells for every 10^8 mouse cells (one spleen) to be fused.
4.	Reimmunize the animals 3–4 days before fusion.
5.	Split myeloma cells 1:1 with fresh medium on the day before fusion.
6.	Fuse cells, plate out in HT medium.
7.	After 24 h, carefully replace the HT medium with HAT medium.
8.	Seven days after fusion feed cells with HT medium.
9.	About 7 days later, refeed with HT medium.
10.	Test supernatants from wells with colonies, as the supernatant turns yellow and the cells are about 50–90 % confluent.
11.	Clone positive wells and refeed with HT medium.
12.	Test clones.
13.	Scale-up and cryopreserve positive clones.

different quality water; the unit used should be intended for tissue culture. When cultures fail to thrive, water quality is often the source of the problem. Medium is conveniently used in 500 ml aliquots and stored at 4 °C before use. Medium should be warmed to 37 °C prior to use. To the medium add 2 mM glutamine, 100 IU ml^{-1} penicillin, 100 mg ml^{-1} streptomycin and fetal bovine serum (FBS) to 10%. If the medium is stored for more than 2 weeks at 4 °C, the levels of the essential amino acid glutamine, and the antibiotics penicillin and streptomycin, should be replenished.

Fetal bovine serum (FBS)

Serum is used to provide additional nutrients to the medium to support cell growth. FBS is still the most commonly used serum additive for tissue culture media. Different batches of FBS support cell growth to different degrees. We screen batches of FBS for ability to support hybridoma growth, although prescreened batches are available commercially. Mixtures of sera have been used for hybridoma culture, and the addition of mouse serum has been reported to increase hybridoma yields. There are a number of variants of calf sera available commercially, some of which are prescreened for hybridoma production. For example, a-gamma (Ig-depleted) calf serum has been shown to produce twice as much immunoglobulin as standard FBS, in both human and mouse hybridoma lines (Torres *et al.*, 1992), and purification of monoclonal antibody subsequently is easier if there is no bovine IgG present. IgG-depleted FBS is available commercially or can be prepared by passing normal calf serum through a protein G column. These replacements for FBS (10% v/v) should be considered only if you encounter problems.

Serum-free media

The risk of introduction of pathogens such as bovine viruses or prions (which cause diseases such as bovine spongiform encephalopathy and

Creutzfeld–Jacob syndrome) and the presence of unwanted proteins in downstream processing has generated the need to use completely defined serum-free medium. Although this is an absolute requirement for therapeutic applications of monoclonal antibodies, it is not always appropriate in research laboratories. The success rate is higher with FBS, and defined media are relatively expensive.

Selection medium

Medium containing hypoxanthine, aminopterin and thymidine (HAT) is used to selectively grow hybrids following fusion. Aminopterin blocks the main biosynthetic pathway for DNA synthesis, while thymidine and hypoxanthine feed the salvage pathways (see Theoretical basis). For each fusion, a fresh bottle of HAT medium should be made by the addition of 100 × stock HAT to the culture medium. You will need about 100 ml of HAT medium/10^8 lymphocytes fused. Medium containing hypoxanthine and thymidine (HT) is used to maintain hybridoma growth. Because hypoxanthine and thymidine are used up by cells in culture whilst aminopterin is not, cells will die unless HT medium is added, until the aminopterin has been diluted out or removed. From 7 days following the fusion, the hybridomas are maintained in medium with HT. Some laboratories wean hybridomas off HT medium once the aminopterin is depleted, but the effort involved outweighs the savings in HT. Stock solutions containing 100 times concentrated HAT or HT are commercially available.

Lysis medium

If spleen cells are used as the source of immune cells for fusion, the erythrocytes are commonly lysed prior to fusion, using isotonic ammonium chloride or Gey's hemolytic medium. However, this step is not essential and can compromise the quality of the lymphocytes.

Polyethylene glycol (PEG)

PEG is the fusion-inducing agent. Batches of PEG vary in their toxicity and ability to induce fusions. PEG should be stored in the dark, to avoid degradation by photooxidation. Some groups add dimethylsulfoxide (DMSO, 15% (v/v)) to the PEG for fusion, but the value of DMSO in the fusion process is questionable. We recommend the use of a commercially available, pretested preparation such as Polyethylene glycol 1500 (Roche Molecular Biochemicals).

4. Screening assay

One of the keys to successful development of a monoclonal antibody is the screening assay. The more specific and simple the screening test, the better the chance of obtaining a monoclonal antibody of interest. The nature of the antigen will often dictate the screening assay. For example, antibodies to surface antigens of cells in suspension can be examined quickly and easily by immunofluorescence (*Chapter 6*), whereas immunoenzyme techniques are suitable for tissue sections and enzyme-linked immunosorbent assay

(ELISA) or radioimmunoassay (RIA) for soluble antigens. The screening method should reflect the techniques in which you wish to use your antibodies. Antibodies that react against fixed tissue will not necessarily react with fresh tissue; some antibodies will work very well in one assay but not in another. It is important to have purified antigen for the assay, since antibodies against impurities in the immunizing material will react if the test material contains the same impurities. The assay must be specific, sensitive and capable of screening large numbers of samples quickly. Appropriate positive and negative controls must be used in every assay. An example of a simple ELISA based screen is described in *Protocol 2.1*, and a typical set of results are shown in *Figure 2.2*.

5. Immunization

Animals can make antibody against a wide range of molecular structures. Animals will usually not make antibody to 'self' antigens, and will not usually recognize small molecules, unless they are conjugated to a carrier molecule. To obtain high affinity IgG antibody, the immunization protocol must invoke T-cell help, which is generally restricted to protein antigens or molecules conjugated to proteins, and requires the germinal center reaction, *in vivo*.

5.1 Selection of antigen

The selection of antigen is critical to the success of antibody generation. As much as 1 mg of antigen may be required for the immunization and screening. The antigen should be as pure as possible because there will be an immune response against contaminants in the preparation. The purity of the antigen used in the detection assay is crucial; methods of screening for antibody against a component of a mixture, such as western immunoblotting or biological assays, are considerably more labor intensive than ELISA. The protein should be no smaller than 3 kDa, and should differ in amino acid sequence from the corresponding endogenous protein, in order to induce an immune response. Smaller or endogenous molecules can be made immunogenic by conjugation to a carrier protein, such as diphtheria toxoid, as described in *Protocol 2.2*.

Synthetic peptides that correspond to an amino acid sequence of the antigen can be prepared or purchased for use as antigen. The peptide should correspond to a sequence that is present on the exterior of the antigen molecule, and should be predicted to be antigenic, on the basis of the literature or antigenicity programs such as MacVector. If the synthetic peptide is small it should be conjugated to a carrier protein (*Protocol 2.2*).

5.2 Standard immunization protocol

There are many protocols for immunization of animals. Generally, antigen in aggregated form is more immunogenic than monomeric protein. The response, especially to soluble antigens is greatly potentiated by using an adjuvant. Complete Freund's adjuvant (CFA) is efficient and still popular, although it is associated with a number of problems. Animal ethics committees are concerned with the side effects of injecting animals with

CFA. Accidental self-injection of minute amounts of adjuvant can cause a painful long-lasting granuloma. Finally, the preparation of a stable antigen/adjuvant emulsion is difficult and unpredictable.

Several adjuvants have been released that are claimed to perform at least as well as CFA, with fewer side effects. We have had very good results with an adjuvant peptide known as GMDP (GERBU™Adjuvant 10, GERBU Biotechnik, Gailberg, Germany) which can be used for multiple boosters because of the absence of adjuvant toxicity.

A 'booster' immunization is commonly given about 2–4 weeks following the primary immunization; this should never be given in CFA because of the risk of anaphylactic shock, but may be given in incomplete Freund's adjuvant (which is the same as CFA except that the mycobacterial component is missing). Preferably, the same aqueous adjuvant as for the primary immunization is used.

A typical immunization protocol for a soluble antigen, available in quantity, is shown in *Figure 2.1* and in *Protocol 2.3*.

Figure 2.2 illustrates a typical range of antibody titers from a conventional immunization regime using a peptide conjugated to diphtheria toxoid. As a rough guide, a titer of greater than 1 in 100 mouse serum is the minimum required to consider using the splenocytes in a fusion. If the mouse was immunized with an impure preparation of antigen and then screened with the same material it is necessary to confirm a specific immune response against the antigen, for example by western blotting to identify the antigen by molecular weight, or by inhibition of the antigen's biological activity.

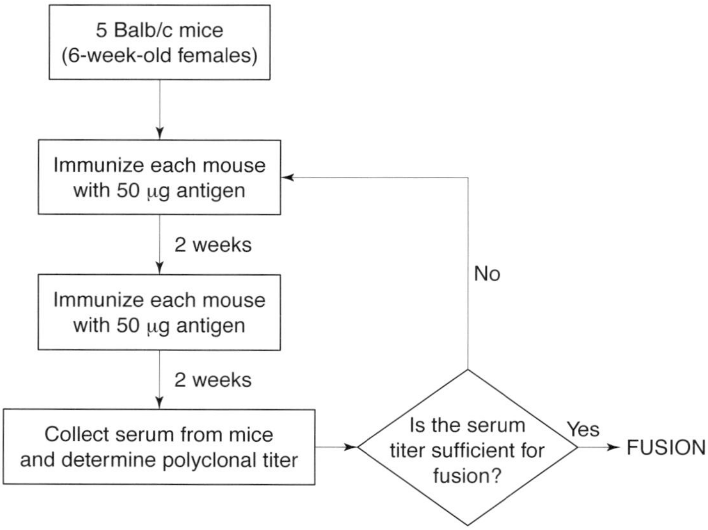

Figure 2.1

Flow diagram for a simple immunization protocol

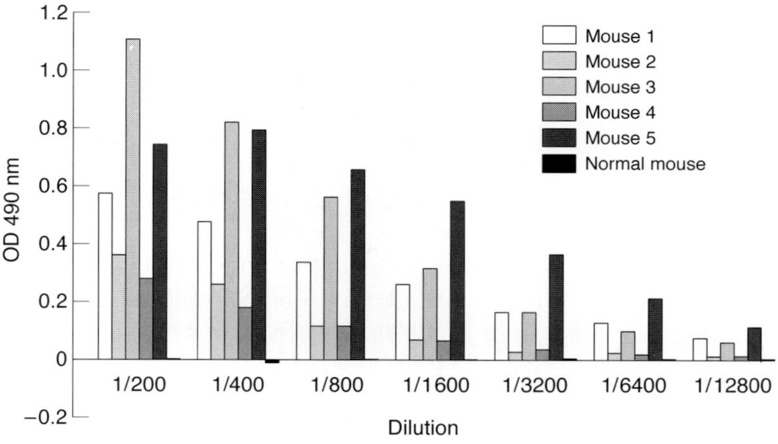

Figure 2.2

Typical polyclonal antiserum dilution curves following conventional immunization of a group of Balb/c mice

5.3 Alternative immunization protocols

Live allogeneic and xenogeneic cells are highly immunogenic, for immunization, typically, cells in saline are injected, intraperitoneally (i.p.), at about 10^7 cells per mouse. A secondary immunization is given four weeks later, 3–4 days prior to fusion, with the same number of cells.

Soluble antigen may be injected intravenously (i.v.), intraperitoneally, subcutaneously (s.c.), or into the foot-pad. All these routes stimulate B cells in the spleen and local lymph nodes, and these are suitable sources of immune B cells. The popliteal lymph nodes are a convenient and rich source of immune cells following foot-pad injection, however, animal ethics committees are increasingly reluctant to allow foot-pad injection. Most work is done with spleen cells.

Low quantities of antigen and poorly soluble antigens cannot be used in conventional immunization protocols as described above. Several techniques have been used to overcome the problems of very low levels of antigen, including *in vitro* immunization, intrasplenic immunization and lymph node deposition. Small amounts of antigen purified on nitrocellulose membranes have been used to immunize animals either by an intrasplenic route or *in vitro*. These methods generally result in monoclonal antibodies of the IgM isotype and often of low affinity.

6. Myeloma cells

A number of myeloma cell lines are available for fusion (*Table 2.2*). In the mouse, where there is the greatest choice and experience, there is no reason for using a line that retains the ability to make its own Ig light or heavy chains, since these will complicate the process of selection of monoclonal

Table 2.2. Mouse myeloma lines widely used for B cell hybridoma production.

Cell line	Reference
SP2/0-Agl4	Shulman *et al.*, 1978
P3-X63-Ag8.653	Kearney *et al.*, 1979
FO	de St. Groth and Scheidegger, 1980
P3-NSI/1-Ag4-1 (secretes kappa chain)	Kohler *et al.*, 1976

hybridomas. A limited amount of work has been done with rat fusions, particularly when making reagents against mouse antigens. These fusions can be done using either rat or mouse myeloma cells as fusion partner. Relatively little work has been done in other species, but the hamster and chicken offer potential advantages. In particular, mammalian Fc receptors do not bind avian Ig strongly, and avian antibodies should therefore show reduced nonspecific binding when used as reagents with mammalian cells.

The maintenance and health of the myeloma fusion partner is of paramount importance in the eventual success of the fusion. Myeloma cells that have been growing for long periods of time or that have been overgrown (i.e. grown to high concentration and partially lost viability) are less successful at producing hybridomas than freshly grown cells. Myeloma cells are thawed from liquid nitrogen just days prior to the fusion procedure. Mycoplasma-contaminated cells have no place in making monoclonal antibodies. Realistically, however, it is nigh impossible to insure that cultures have not become contaminated since the last mycoplasma screening test. If you have cell lines that grow more slowly than usual, that appear to change the medium pH rapidly, or develop unusual growth characteristics, there is a good chance that mycoplasma infection has occurred. Throw the cells out together with frozen stocks from the same batch.

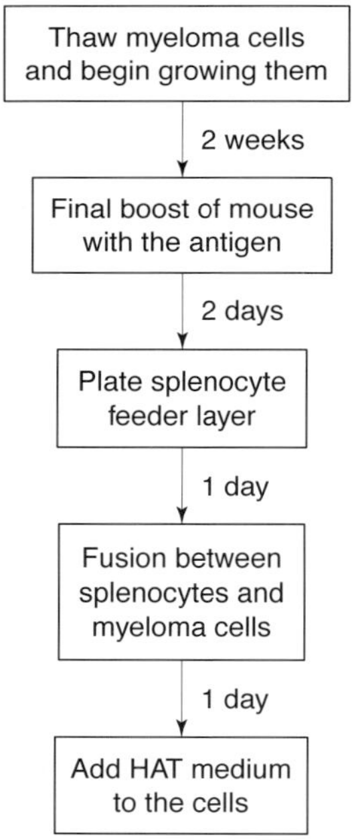

Figure 2.3

Flow diagram of the major steps required to accomplish a successful fusion between B lymphocyte from an immunized mouse and myeloma cells

7. Fusion protocol

The established fusion protocols use PEG to induce membrane fusion. Electroporation and electroacoustic techniques are alternatives that are especially useful when low numbers of specific B cells are available for fusion. When combined with *in vitro* immunization methods, the purification of antigen-specific B cells followed by electroporation enables the production of monoclonal antibodies against low amounts of antigen. These specialized methods are not described here.

There are many variations of the 'standard' fusion protocol. The one described in *Figure 2.3* and *Protocol 2.4* is used in the authors' laboratory to produce monoclonal antibodies against a variety of antigens ranging from cell surface antigens to soluble proteins.

8. Post-fusion care

Seven days after plating out the cells in HAT medium, replace half the medium with fresh medium containing HT, instead of HAT. At this time, small colonies of hybridoma cells may be visible. As the colonies grow, withdraw medium and test for antibody activity in the screening assay. Replace medium in the wells with fresh HT medium, as the medium becomes acidic (yellow). This can be a busy time, and the benefits of a solid screening assay will soon become apparent! The stages associated with this part of the procedure are summarized in *Figure 2.4*. It is important to inspect the wells under a microscope every day. Hybridomas are fast growing and once in exponential phase growth they can quickly deplete the glucose.

When the cells have expanded to cover half of the well bottom and the medium begins to turn orange the cultures are ready for screening. After collecting a sample for screening, the remaining medium is aspirated from the well and replaced with fresh medium. If a well tests positive for antibody activity, the cells should be quickly expanded and cloned. It is

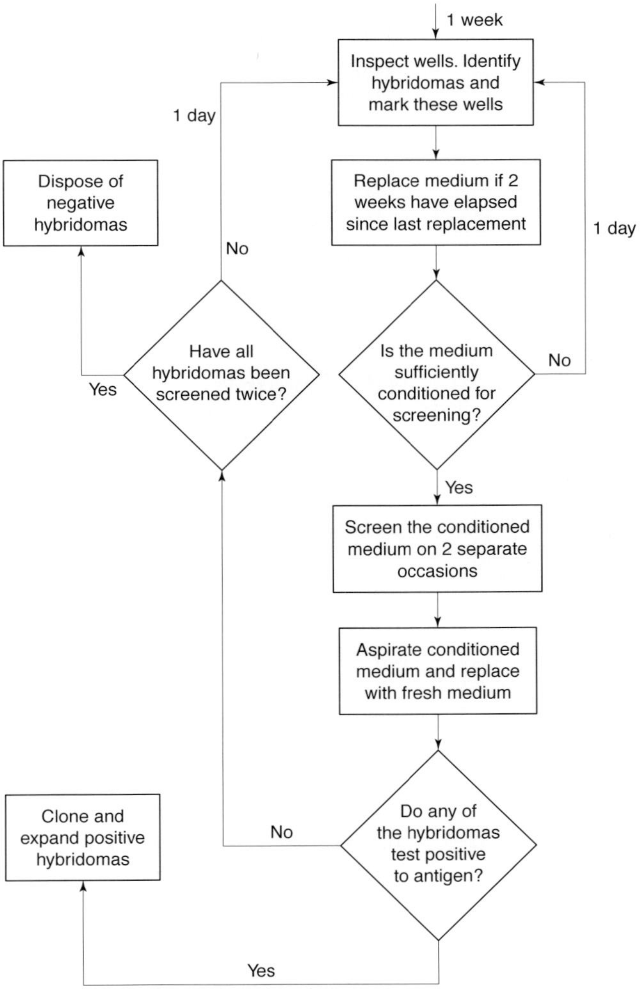

Figure 2.4

Summary of postfusion procedures

possible for two different hybridomas to inhabit the same well. If one secretes antibody and the other does not the potential exists for the faster growing nonsecretor to out-compete the secretor. This is avoided by cloning the cells from the positive well early. When the medium is sufficiently conditioned it is retested. If the medium tests positive this is confirmation of antibody activity. The term conditioned, as used in this context, refers to the results of cell growth, which alter the medium by utilizing nutrients, changing pH, producing waste materials and frequently growth factors and, in the case of hybridomas, antibody.

9. Cloning

Once the screening assay indicates that a well contains an antibody of interest, the contents of the well should be cloned as soon as possible. It is important to clone positive wells so as to prevent them being overgrown by negative clones, and to avoid working with mixed clones. While there are several cloning methods, the most common is that of limiting dilution. The rationale behind cloning is to plate out cells from a starting culture into a number of individual wells so that the most probable number of cells in any given well is one. According to Poisson's distribution, if the probable cell number per well is one, then 37% of wells will have no cells, and hence no growth. However, because the cloning efficiency may be less than one, it is advisable to clone at predicted frequencies of both one and three cells per well, and to plate out 96 wells per concentration. Cloning is described in *Protocol 2.5*.

10. Cryopreservation

Preserving cells in liquid nitrogen is the only means of ensuring the long-term availability of hybridomas. Cells should be frozen down as soon as possible and a detailed record kept of what the cells are and when they were stored. We make a Master Cell Bank containing at least ten vials of each line, frozen on at least two separate occasions. If possible, arrange for a second set of vials to be stored in an independent laboratory. While there are a number of commercially available controlled-rate freezing systems, the simple system described in *Protocol 2.7* is adequate.

11. Specificity and isotyping

Once the monoclonal antibody has been generated and safeguarded by the establishment of a cell bank, the specificity and the immunoglobulin isotype should be determined. If the antigen is a pure protein, the specificity can usually be determined by measuring its activity against as many closely related proteins as possible using the initial screening assay. If the antigen is a component of an impure preparation, Western blotting, as described in *Chapter 4*, may help to establish the specificity of the monoclonal antibody.

Antibody isotyping ELISA kits are commercially available. They can screen for the classes IgA, IgM and the subclasses of IgG and are easy to use according to the manufacturer's instructions.

12. Mycoplasma

Mycoplasma contamination may be detected by a number of methods, including staining with fluorescent DNA-binding dyes, monoclonal antibody or cDNA probes. The well established dye methods are effective and straightforward in use; dyes and instructions on interpretation are available from tissue culture suppliers. A polymerase chain reaction (PCR) method gives improved specificity and sensitivity.

The aim of identification of mycoplasma infection is to eliminate the source rather than save a particular culture. It is possible to cure contaminated cultures of mycoplasma infection, but this should be attempted only if there is no back-up source of uncontaminated cells. The most effective way to eliminate mycoplasma is to passage the cells through mice. *In vitro* 'curing' of mycoplasma infection, using antibiotics or antibody may be effective, but it is difficult to be sure that the mycoplasma have been eliminated completely. They may grow back, and the result may be contamination of other cultures. Mycoplasma cure should be reserved for unique hybridomas and should not be applied to the fusion partner, because if cure is not complete the problem will inevitably return in hybridomas derived from the fusion. It is usually possible to get fresh, uncontaminated stock of the fusion partner from another laboratory.

13. Large scale antibody production

13.1 Ascitic fluid

The generation of ascites tumours in mice was widely used to produce large quantities of monoclonal antibodies. Technically this is a straightforward and economical production method yielding from 0.5 to 5 mg Ig ml^{-1}; with the costs depending to a large extent on local animal house charges. However, ascites production can not be justified ethically when alternative methods of producing large quantities of monoclonal antibody exist.

13.2 Cell Factory

The simplest alternative to ascitic fluid production is the use of the Cell Factory such as that produced by Nunc. The Cell Factory is essentially a large tissue culture flask divided into many levels in order to increase the surface area available for cell adhesion. The cell density is typical of other tissue culture flasks and therefore growth medium containing 10% serum is required. The major disadvantage is that large volumes of dilute antibody must be collected for purification but high cell densities can be achieved and maintained for many months, if required, allowing production of substantial quantities of antibody with minimum expense and effort.

13.3 Perfusion cell culture

The large-scale production of monoclonal antibodies is now feasible for most laboratories already engaged in hybridoma production. There is a range of continuous perfusion systems or 'mini-bioreactors' from single disposable units producing 300–1000 mg per month to pilot scale systems producing up to 10 g per month. For the short-term user a single disposable unit requiring only a small peristaltic pump may be convenient.

Widely used cell culture systems include Cell Pharm (UniSyn Technologies, Tustin, CA, USA), miniPerm (Heraeus Instruments, Osterode am Harz, Germany) and CellMax (Cellco Inc., Germantown, MD, USA). While there are differences in these systems, the basic principle is the same. Each bioreactor has a large number of hollow fibers packed within a silicone membrane. Cells are cultured at high densities within the extra-capillary spaces and receive a constant supply of nutrients pumped through the hollow fibers. Waste products are removed from the system via the hollow fibers. The hollow fibers have a pore size cut off of 10 000–70 000 allowing the passage of the required nutrients, but retaining serum and the antibodies produced in the extra-capillary space. This has the additional advantage of being economical on serum, requiring less than 10 ml per month for a single small cartridge. A sufficient oxygen supply is maintained by the passage of air across the silicone membrane.

The smaller units are maintained in a standard CO_2 incubator and require a peristaltic pump to move the medium through the system. The larger systems have their own incubator and pump with computerized controls. The middle of the range systems consist of a number of mini-bioreactors in parallel, fed from a single unit which can have a programmable flow rate. As the cells and antibodies are kept in the extra-capillary space, it is possible to have a number of cell lines growing in separate cartridges at the same time.

The high cell density results in a high concentration of endogenous growth factors. Consequently the proportion of serum in the growth medium may be reduced without a decrease in metabolic activity.

Conditioned medium of high antibody concentration can be harvested periodically. In the experience of the authors, with a CellMax system, approximately 80% of the antibody is retained on the outside of the capillaries. In return for the initial expense of purchasing the pump and artificial capillary module, it is possible to produce 7 mg/day of antibody indefinitely and the small volumes of highly concentrated antibody in the conditioned medium are easy to purify with Protein G affinity chromatography.

The nutrient requirements of cell lines in bioreactors are somewhat different to those of cells in standard tissue culture conditions. In particular, the rate of glucose metabolism is greatly increased and it is advisable to monitor glucose. Monitoring the pH is not reliable for these culture systems, as we have found that the medium has been depleted of glucose long before the medium changes color. This is particularly critical during the initial period in the bioreactor. Additional glucose may be added to the medium; however, the osmolarity of the medium may need to be adjusted accordingly. The next generation of bioreactors is likely to include a constant glucose monitor. Unisyn Technologies now market a specially formulated medium for use in hollow-fiber bioreactors, incorporating higher concentrations of glucose and glutamine.

Some of the systems allow a number of units to be used in parallel; and do not require that they all be set up at the one time. Whilst this is convenient, the units will all have to run at a single flow rate which may not be optimal for all lines. One particular concern is the ever present threat of contamination. It is vital that all media and cell lines are checked for contaminants as rigorously as possible.

Further information on the specifics of individual systems can be obtained from the suppliers. Before embarking on the use of one of these systems, it would be advisable to confer with the suppliers and particularly with current users.

14. Antibody purification

Although there are numerous methods available to purify monoclonal antibodies, in most cases a one step affinity purification of the antibody is acceptable, although for therapeutic application of monoclonal antibodies at least two purification steps are required by regulatory authorities.

The purification needed depends on the use to which the antibody will be put. In many instances, culture supernatant containing the desired antibody may be adequate. When the antibody is to be labelled, or used as a reagent for purification of the antigen, it needs to be purified. The antibody class and concentration must be determined in order to decide what method is most likely to work. Antibody class can be determined using a variety of commercial kits, based on specific antibodies against the Ig isotypes. The percentage yield and purity of antibody should be determined after purification, to assess the suitability of the method selected.

14.1 Precipitation

Purification methods can be divided into two broad categories: precipitation methods and chromatographic methods. Precipitation methods can either remove the unwanted components, leaving the antibody in solution, as with caprylic acid or Rivanol, or precipitate the antibodies, as with PEG or saturated ammonium sulfate (SAS). These techniques will enrich not only the required antibody but also other immunoglobulins present in either ascites fluid or culture supernatant containing serum.

14.2 Chromatography

A widely used approach combines preliminary enrichment with PEG or SAS with final fractionation by chromatography. Chromatographic processes for monoclonal antibody purification include protein A, protein G, ion exchange, hydroxylapatite and thiophilic adsorption chromatography. Many of these procedures have been adapted for high-pressure liquid chromatography (HPLC) (Abe and Inouye, 1993). For a detailed discussion on the purification of monoclonal antibodies using chromatographic procedures see Nau (1989) and Strickler and Gemski (1987).

No one procedure, or combination of procedures, is suitable for all monoclonal antibodies. While purification of IgG antibodies is straightforward, IgM antibodies are more challenging. HPLC on hydroxylapatite has been useful in obtaining purified IgG and, to a lesser extent, IgM. Hydroxylapatite coated onto ceramic beads (Macroprep Ceramic HPHT, Bio-Rad, Richmond, CA, USA) has been successful for IgM purification. Hydroxylapatite chromatography does not require low pH to elute the purified antibodies, unlike protein A and protein G. Acid elution may affect the long-term stability of antibodies.

When embarking on purification, do not commit all your antibody in one go. There may have to be a choice between having adequate amounts of antibody with some impurities and having very small amounts of high purity material. Bear in mind that low concentrations of highly pure antibody have a tendency to 'disappear' by adsorbing on to the surfaces of the vessels in which they are stored.

14.3 Protein G

The single most useful purification procedure for monoclonal antibodies is affinity purification on protein G. It is a simple procedure and requires minimal equipment (although a UV monitor at 280 nm is helpful). If treated carefully, a protein G column can last for a considerable length of time and will pay for itself many times over. In addition, purification by affinity methods has the advantage of concentrating the antibodies. This can be particularly useful when large volumes of culture supernatant containing low concentrations of antibody are involved. At a pH between 6.0 and 8.0 the Fc portions of all subclasses of IgG are bound to the protein G matrix. Once all the crude antibody has been applied to the column and it has been washed with a number of column volumes of loading buffer, the purified antibody can be eluted from the column with buffer at a pH ranging from 4 to 2. The protein G can be packed into a syringe barrel with a glass wool plug at the bottom.

We use ProSep G™ protein G (Bioprocessing Ltd., Durham, UK). Ten ml of the adsorbent binds approximately 80 mg of monoclonal antibody before high levels of antibody are detected in the column flow through. *Protocol 2.7* describes the procedure for an IgG_1 subclass monoclonal antibody. Other subclasses may elute under different conditions. Citric acid of pH in the range 2–5 should be tried, beginning with the highest pH. If a high pH eluent is effective there is no need to use a more acid eluent, which may denature the monoclonal antibody irreversibly.

15. Storage and quality control

Once the final antibody characteristics have been determined and the protein concentration is known, the antibody should be dispensed and stored as appropriate. This will depend on the final use of the antibody but we tend to aliquot the antibody into vials after the dialysis step and then freeze-dry from the dialysis buffer without further addition. Sometimes, preservatives and bulking agents such as mannitol are added but care should be taken as the use of sodium azide as a preservative is not compatible with many immunocytochemical and functional applications of monoclonal antibodies.

The final step is one of quality control to establish that freeze-drying and storage have not altered the antibody. We normally set up a stability protocol consisting of the screening assay, a protein assay and one other measurement such as a gel, to determine common identity and characteristics of each batch of antibody.

Further reading

Campbell, A.M. (1991) *Monoclonal Antibody and Immunosensor Technology: Laboratory Techniques in Biochemistry and Molecular Biology*. Elsevier Science, Amsterdam.

Langone, J.J. and van Vunakis, H. (1983) *Methods in Enzymology, Vol. 92 Immunochemical Techniques*. Academic Press, Orlando, FL.

Goding, J.W. (1996) *Monoclonal Antibodies: Principles and Practice*. 3rd edn. Academic Press, London.

Peters, J.U. and Baumgarten, H. (1992) *Monoclonal Antibodies*. Springer-Verlag, New York.

Schook, L.B. (1987) *Monoclonal Antibody Production Techniques and Applications*. Marcel Dekker Inc., New York.

Weir, D.M., Herzenberg, L.A. and Blackwell, C. (1986) *Handbook of Experimental Immunology, Vol. 4: Applications of Immunological Methods in the Biomedical Sciences*, 4th edn. Blackwell Scientific Publications, Oxford.

Zola, H. (1987) *Monoclonal Antibodies: A Manual of Techniques*. CRC Press, Boca Raton, FL.

References

Abe, N. and Inouye, K. (1993) Purification of monoclonal antibodies with light-chain heterogeneity produced by mouse hybridomas raised with NS-1 myelomas: application of hydrophobic interaction high-performance liquid chromatography. *J. Biochem. Biophys. Methods* **27**, 215–227.

de St Groth, S.F. and Scheidegger, D. (1980) Production of monoclonal antibodies: strategy and tactics. *J. Immunol. Methods* **35**, 1–21.

Freshney, R.I. (1983) *Culture of Animal Cells: A Manual of Basic Technique*. Alan R. Liss Inc., New York.

Kearney, J.F., Radbruch, A., Liesegang, B. and Rajewsky, K. (1979) A new mouse myeloma cell line that has lost immunoglobulin expression but permits the construction of antibody-secreting hybrid cell lines. *J. Immunol.* **123**, 1548–1550.

King, L.B. and Ashwell, J.D. (1993) Signalling for death of lymphoid cells. *Curr. Opin. Immunol.* **5**, 368–373.

Kohler, G. and Milstein, C. (1975) Continuous cultures of fused cells secreting antibody of predefined specificity. *Nature* **256**, 495–497.

Kohler, G., Howe, S.C. and Milstein, C. (1976) Fusion between immunoglobulin-secreting and non-secreting myeloma cell lines. *Eur. J. Immunol.* **6**, 292–295.

Nau, D.R. (1989) Chromatographic methods for antibody purification and analysis. *BioChromatography*, **4**, 4–18.

Shulman, M., Wilde, C.D. and Kohler, G. (1978) A better cell line for making hybridomas secreting specific antibodies. *Nature* **276**, 269–270.

Strickler, M.P. and Gemski, M.J. (1987) Single-step purification of monoclonal antibodies by anion exchange chromatography high-performance liquid chromatography. In: *Commercial Production of Monoclonal Antibodies*, pp. 217–245 (Seaver, S.S., ed.). Marcel Dekker Inc., New York.

Torres, A.R., Healey, M.C., Johnston, A.V. and McKnight, M.E. (1992) Growth of hybridoma cells and antibody production in a gamma calf serum. *Hum. Antibod. Hybrid.* **3**, 206–211.

Protocol 2.1

Screening hybridomas by enzyme-linked immunoassay (ELISA)

Equipment

96 multiwell microtiter ELISA plates

ELISA plate reader with a 490 nm optical filter

Multichannel pipette

Reagents

5 μg of antigen per ELISA plate

Bovine serum albumin

Horseradish peroxidase conjugated rabbit antimouse immunoglobulin (or IgG) antibody

Coating buffer: 0.795 g Na_2CO_3, 1.465 g $NaHCO_3$, 500 ml MilliQ-purified water. Adjust pH to 9.6 with HCl or NaOH as necessary

Washing buffer: 146.1 g NaCl, 1.0 g KH_2PO_4, 4.6 g Na_2HPO_4, 2.5 ml Tween 20, 5 l MilliQ-purified water. Adjust pH to 7.6 with HCl or NaOH as necessary

Substrate buffer: 3.65 g citric acid monohydrate, 4.755 g Na_2HPO_4, 500 ml MilliQ purified water. Adjust pH to 5.0 with HCl or NaOH as necessary

Ortho-phenylene diamine (OPD) solution: 0.01 g OPD, 10 ml 30% (w/v) hydrogen peroxide solution, 10 ml substrate buffer

Protocol

1. Dilute the antigen to 1 μg ml^{-1} in coating buffer. Use the multichannel pipette to deliver 100 μl to each well on one half of the plate, and 100 μl of coating buffer alone to each well on the other half of the plate. Cover the plate with parafilm and place in an incubator at 37°C for 3 h.
2. Prepare a blocking solution of 2% (w/v) bovine serum albumin (BSA) in washing buffer. Empty the wells and fill to the top with washing buffer. Empty the washing buffer. Wash the plate four times. Dispense 100 μl of the blocking solution per well. Cover the plate with parafilm and place in a refrigerator at 4°C overnight. The next day, wash the plates four times.
3. Prepare appropriate dilutions of the test solution (either mouse serum or hybridoma medium) in Dulbecco's phosphate buffered saline (DPBS). Include serum from a normal mouse or medium as a negative control. Include a positive control (i.e. pre-existing antibody) if available. Deliver serial dilutions of each sample in DPBS in triplicate (100 μl per well) to the antigen side and to the control side of the plate. Incubate at 37°C for 3 h.

4. Wash the plates six times and add 100 μl of horseradish peroxidase conjugated rabbit anti-mouse immunoglobulin antibody, diluted 1:2000 in 0.5% BSA in wash buffer, to each well. Incubate the plates at 37°C for 90 min, and wash six times. Add 100 μl of OPD solution per well and incubate at 37°C for 30 min. Stop the enzyme reaction with 50 μl of 1M sulfuric acid per well.

5. Measure the optical density of the wells at 490 nm with an ELISA plate reader. Determine the titer by subtracting the optical density of the uncoated wells from the optical density of the antigen coated wells, after importing the data to a spreadsheet such as Excel or Lotus. Plot the optical density as a function of dilution.

Protocol 2.2

Conjugation of antigen to a carrier protein

Materials

Carrier protein (e.g. diphtheria toxoid). The mass ratio of carrier protein to antigen should be 4 : 1

Glutaraldehyde solution (0.13 M)

Dialysis membrane with a molecular weight cut off that will allow unconjugated hapten to dialyse out but retain conjugate.

TBS buffer (Tris base, 0.1 M; NaCl, 0.15 M, pH 8)

Protocol

1. Dilute the antigen to a concentration of 2.5 mg ml^{-1} in TBS.
2. Dilute carrier protein to a concentration of 2 mg ml^{-1} in TBS.
3. Mix carrier and protein in 4 : 1 mass ratio in a beaker with a magnetic stirring bar.
4. Add glutaraldehyde solution 1 volume per 2.4 volumes of protein solution. Add the glutaraldehyde solution to the continuously stirred protein over a period of 20 min and continue stirring for 90 min at room temperature.
5. Dialyse the reaction mixture against 2000 volumes of TBS for 16 h at 4°C.

Protocol 2.3

Immunization with a soluble protein available in quantity

Materials

5 six-week old female Balb/c mice

Approximately 250 μg of the antigen

Sterile isotonic saline or phosphate buffered saline pH 7

10 μg vial of GMPD adjuvant (GERBU™ Adjuvant 10, GERBU Biotechnik, GmbH, Gailberg, Germany)

1 ml syringe and a 27 gauge injection needle

Protocol

1. Resuspend 250 μg of the antigen in 1 ml of the aqueous solution.
2. Transfer the resuspended antigen to a 10 μg vial of GERBU™ adjuvant and agitate to dissolve the adjuvant.
3. Take the antigen into a 1 ml syringe. Tap the syringe with the nozzle facing upwards in order to dislodge bubbles from the internal surface of the syringe. Attach the needle to the syringe and depress the piston to check that the solution flows through the needle.
4. A single injection of 200 μl of the solution is made into the intraperitoneal cavity.

Note

Check on the welfare of the mice on a regular basis. Any distressed mice must be euthanased. This procedure can be repeated as often as required until an appropriate antiserum titer is obtained in at least one of the mice. Bleeding of mice should be carried out by, or under the instruction of, a skilled animal technician.

Protocol 2.4

Fusion – standard protocol using polyethylene glycol (PEG)

Equipment

Sterile scissors and forceps to remove the spleen

Sterile loose fitting teflon glass homogenizer

Bench-top centrifuge

Hemocytometer

Timer

Petri dish

10 × 24 well flat-bottomed culture plates

Reagents

250 ml of pre-warmed Dulbecco's phosphate buffered saline (DPBS) containing 2% (w/v) fetal bovine serum (FBS)

Trypan blue

250 ml of pre-warmed DMEM with the addition of 20% (v/v) FBS and 100 mM hypoxanthine and 16 mM thymidine (HT-media supplement)

250 ml of pre-warmed DMEM with 20% (v/v) FBS, and 100 mM hypoxanthine and 16 mM thymidine (HT)

Prewarmed polyethylene glycol (PEG 1500) solution (commercial preparation, see *Section 3.2*)

250 ml pre-warmed DMEM

500 ml prewarmed DMEM with 20% (v/v) FBS, and 100 mM hypoxanthine, 400 mM aminopterin and 16 mM thymidine (HAT)

250 ml prewarmed DPBS

Myeloma cells

Immunized mouse. The animal determined as the best responder is boosted 3 days before the fusion so that the population of antibody-secreting B lymphocytes is also in log growth phase at the time of the fusion.

Normal mouse as source of feeder cells, or hybridoma growth factor (for example Hybridoma Fusion and Cloning Supplement, from Boehringer Mannheim).

Protocol Part A – Preparation of spleen cells

1. Kill the mouse by CO_2 inhalation and remove the spleen aseptically (soak the mouse in 70% ethanol prior to opening the peritoneal cavity). Pull the skin

tight over the abdomen with forceps and use the scissors to cut the skin from the abdomen to reveal an area of peritoneum 3 cm in diameter. Make an incision and remove the spleen by cutting away connective tissue.

2. Transfer the spleen into a petri dish containing DPBS-2% FBS and trim any remaining fat. Make incisions in the spleen to hasten its disintegration when homogenized.
3. Place 10 ml of DPBS-2% FBS in the homogenizer. Transfer the spleen and use a loose-fitting piston to form a uniform suspension of splenocytes. Transfer the cell suspension to a centrifuge tube. Wash the homogenizer with 10 ml of DPBS-2% FBS to transfer the remaining cells to the centrifuge tube. Remove the spleen capsule from the suspension.
4. Centrifuge the cell suspension at 90 g for 3 min. Aspirate the supernatant and resuspend the cells in 10 ml DPBS without FBS. Centrifuge again, and resuspend the cells in 10 ml serum-free DMEM. Count the number of viable cells with the hemocytometer, using Trypan blue dye to stain dead cells.

Protocol part B – Myeloma cell preparation

1. About 2 weeks before fusion day thaw out myeloma cells and establish in culture in DMEM-10% FBS. You will need four 150 cm^2 flasks for fusion with cells from one mouse spleen.
2. On the fusion day examine the myeloma cells and perform a cell count; if the viability is less than 80%, postpone the fusion. Approximately 10^8 to 3×10^8 cells are required. Transfer the myeloma cells to centrifuge tubes and spin at 90 g for 3 min. Aspirate the supernatant. Resuspend the cells in DPBS and spin as before. Remove the supernatant and resuspend the cells in 10 ml serum-free DMEM. Count the number of viable cells with the hemocytometer.

Protocol part C – Fusion

1. Place the PEG in a water bath heated to 37°C.
2. Mix equal numbers of myeloma cells and splenocytes in a 50 ml centrifuge tube. Typically 10^8 to 3×10^8 splenocytes are extracted from one spleen. Centrifuge at 90 g for 3 min. Aspirate the supernatant.
3. Add 1 ml of prewarmed PEG to the cell pellet and slowly agitate the suspension in the water bath. Simultaneously start the timer. After 1 minute has elapsed add 7 ml of serum-free DMEM dropwise at the rate of 1 ml per minute. It is important that the PEG1500 be diluted slowly, otherwise osmotic shock damages the cells.
4. After a total of 8 min carefully add 8 ml of DMEM-20% FBS-HT. Centrifuge the suspension at 40 g for 10 min. Aspirate the supernatant and resuspend the cell pellet gently in 250 ml of DMEM-20% FBS-HT.
5. Seed control wells of the plates prepared with a feeder layer the previous day (alternatively, add Hybridoma Fusion and Cloning Medium, Boehringer Mannheim to the culture medium and dispense with feeder cells). Add 1 ml

of the myeloma cell suspension to each of five control wells and 1 ml of the splenocyte suspension to each of five control wells, taking care not to disturb the feeder layer. Splenocytes and myeloma cells are seeded at the same density as the wells containing fused cells, in DMEM-20% FBS-HT.

6. Add 1 ml of the fused cell suspension to each of the other wells. Place the plated cells in an incubator at 37°C with an atmosphere of 5% CO_2.
7. After 24 h, very carefully aspirate the medium from the wells and dispense 2 ml per well of DMEM-20% FBS-HAT.

Notes

The feeder layer cells provide essential growth factors to hybridomas after fusion. Improved yields of hybridomas are obtained by the addition of feeder cells or growth factors. The active ingredient of hybridoma growth factors is probably interleukin-6 (IL-6), the addition of which can increase the yield of monoclonal antibodies. A variant of the Sp2/0 myeloma, transfected so that it produces IL-6, is reported to improve hybridoma yields by up to 15-fold (King and Ashwell, 1993). In the absence of IL-6 or the Sp2/0 variant, add feeder cells. Feeders can be murine thymocytes, spleen cells, peritoneal wash-out cells from a non-immunized mouse or mixed thymocyte conditioned medium prepared from rat thymus. The feeder cells are added to the wells (1 ml) to be used for the fusion products 1 day before the fusion and are cultured under normal conditions.

When killing the mouse, remember to obtain a blood sample and prepare the serum to determine the final polyclonal antibody titer and to use as a positive control in screening.

Different brands of cell culture plates vary in their ability to yield hybridomas; we use plates from COSTAR.

Note that if the piston is tight the cells will be disrupted.

The fusion technique, with practice, takes about 2 hours. Two people working together can prepare the splenocytes and the myeloma cells in parallel.

Resuspending the cells and plating out should be done gently and slowly, using pipettes with wide bores, because at this stage the cell fusion products are susceptible to damage by shear forces. If the cell pellet cannot be resuspended following the centrifugation step, then one of two things has gone wrong. Either the mixing on addition of the PEG was insufficient or the centrifugation step was too hard. In either case the fusion will give a very low yield and it is now time to repeat the procedure on the backup mouse.

There appears to be an advantage to seeding in media containing HT, allowing the cells to recover fully from the fusion before applying the selection medium containing aminopterin.

Protocol 2.5

Cloning of hybridoma cells

Materials

96-well, flat-bottomed tissue culture plates

500 ml of HT medium

Protocol

1. If there is a single colony present in the well, this can be taken out and placed into a new well. Usually, however, a single colony cannot be distinguished. In this case, mix the contents of the well by gentle pipetting and transfer the contents to a new well.
2. Count the harvested cells, prepare suspensions at 30 and 10 cells ml^{-1} in 10 ml of HT medium, and plate the mixture into 96-well, flat-bottomed microtiter plates at 100 μl/well.
3. After 7 days add 100 μl of HT medium to each well.
4. When colonies are seen and the medium begins to go yellow (normally within 5–14 days), test the supernatant from wells containing single colonies and, if positive, scale-up the cultures.

Hints and tips

After removing cells for cloning, feed the cells remaining in the well with HT medium, allow them to proliferate and cryopreserve as soon as possible, to act as a back-up should the cloned cells not survive.

Protocol 2.6

Cryopreservation of hybridoma cells

Materials

Approximately 5×10^7 hybridoma cells in exponential phase growth

Sterile dimethyl sulfoxide (DMSO)

Fetal bovine serum (FBS)

10 plastic cryovials

2 halves of a polystyrene tube rack

Hemocytometer

Trypan blue

Protocol

1. Vigorously agitate the tissue culture flasks to detach the cells. Transfer the cell suspension into 50 ml centrifuge tubes.
2. Take small aliquots and count the cells with the hemocytometer.
3. Centrifuge at 90 **g** for 5 min.
4. Calculate the number of cryovials and the volume of freezing medium that will be required; aim to resuspend 5×10^6 hybridoma cells in 0.5 ml of freezing medium for each vial. For 10 cryovials, prepare the freezing medium by adding 0.5 ml of DMSO to 4.5 ml of FBS.
5. Aspirate the supernatant and resuspend the cells in 5 ml of freezing medium. Place 0.5 ml of cell suspension into each vial.
6. Place the cryovials into 1 half of a polystyrene tube rack and completely enclose the vials with the other half of the rack. Tape the two halves together and leave them overnight in a –80°C freezer.
7. The next day transfer the cryovials to liquid nitrogen tanks.
8. Within a few days, thaw out one vial to check that the cells survived the freezing process. Place the vial in a water bath at 37°C. As soon as the ice has melted, transfer the cell suspension to a 75 cm^2 tissue culture flask containing 20 ml of growth medium.
9. Inspect the cells under a microscope the next day to determine viability.

Hints and tips

Cell viability is preserved by freezing gradually and by thawing quickly.

Wear a face shield when using liquid nitrogen. Vials can explode when being thawed.

Individual hybridomas can be quite different in their growth characteristics; adequate records will ensure that thawed lines are treated in the optimal manner.

Protocol 2.7

Purification of IgG1 on Protein G

Equipment

Small chromatography column (internal diameter 10 mm)

Positive displacement pump

UV absorbance detector and Chart recorder

Fraction collector

Sample loop (40 μl)

Materials

10 ml of Prosep-G affinity adsorbent

Dialysis tubing (molecular weight cut-off 3.5 kDa)

Loading buffer: 1.19 g Na_2HPO_4 (anhydrous), 0.2 g KH_2PO_4, 0.2 g KCl, 8.0 g NaCl, 37.5 g glycine, 1 l MilliQ-purified water. Adjust pH to 7.4 with HCl or NaOH as necessary

Washing buffer: 21 g citric acid monohydrate, 1 l MilliQ-purified water. Adjust pH to 5.0 with HCl or NaOH as necessary

Elution buffer: 21 g Citric acid monohydrate, 1 l MilliQ-purified water. Adjust pH to 2.0 with HCl

Regeneration buffer: hydrochloric acid (1 M) pH 1.5

Dialysis buffer: 11.9 g Na_2HPO_4, 2.0 g KH_2PO_4, 0.2 g KCl, 8.0 g NaCl, 1 l MilliQ-purified water. Adjust pH to 7.4 with HCl or NaOH as necessary

Storage buffer: As for loading buffer but add 0.02% (w/w) sodium azide

Protocol

1. Centrifuge the conditioned growth medium at 90 g for 5 min to remove the cells. Collect the supernatant.
2. Filter the supernatant through a 0.45 μm sterile membrane.
3. Pack the column with affinity adsorbent.
4. Degas buffers by filtering under negative pressure through 0.22 μm membranes before use.
5. Equilibrate the column with loading buffer at a flow rate of 2 ml min^{-1} and monitor the UV absorbance at 214 or 280 nm. Maintain the buffer flow until a baseline is obtained. Begin a flow rate of elution buffer and continue until a baseline is similarly obtained.

6. Inject the conditioned medium in to the sample loop. The binding capacity of the column is approximately 80 mg of monoclonal antibody.
7. Load the conditioned medium on to the column at 2 ml min^{-1}. Collect the column effluent.
8. Once the medium has finished loading begin a 2 ml min^{-1} flow of loading buffer. Maintain the buffer flow until UV absorbance baseline is attained.
9. Wash the column with washing buffer at 2 ml min^{-1}. Maintain the buffer flow until UV absorbance baseline is attained.
10. Begin a 2 ml min^{-1} flow of elution buffer through the adsorbent. As soon as the absorbance peak starts, begin collecting the effluent. Continue eluting until the UV absorbance baseline is attained.
11. Begin a 2 ml min^{-1} flow of regenerating buffer through the column. As soon as the absorbance peak starts, begin collecting the effluent. Continue regenerating until the UV absorbance baseline is attained. In the authors' experience some monoclonal antibody elutes in the regenerating buffer and it is advisable to collect this fraction.
12. Equilibrate the column with storage buffer and store the column at 4°C.
13. Pour the pools into two separate sections of dialysis tubing. Tie off the ends and clamp to insure there is no leakage. Place the dialysis tubing into 1 l of dialysis buffer. Stir at 4°C overnight. It is best to dialyze the pools immediately after collection as long-term incubation with the elution buffer denatures the monoclonal antibody.
14. As a precaution to minimize the risk of microbial contamination, filter the dialyzed antibody through a 0.22 μm membrane prior to storage. Freezing monoclonal antibody to –20°C and then thawing can result in a 50% loss in titer. It is suggested that antibody be stored at 4°C.
15. Assay a sample of the original conditioned medium, the flow through, the eluted peaks and any peak eluted during regeneration. The aim is to calculate the proportion of antibody loaded that appears in the flow through. If a significant proportion of the antibody appears in the flow through it should be reloaded and purified.
16. Run a gel of the antibody preparation under reducing conditions. Visualize the protein bands with Coomassie Blue staining. Under reducing conditions, two separate bands are observed which correspond to the heavy and light chains of the antibody. The gel should indicate the purity of the antibody. If the purification is effective at least 95% of the protein is antibody. The protein concentration of the antibody preparation may be determined using a commercial protein assay kit.

The Basics

Chapter 3

Antibody engineering

M A Thiel, G Pilkington and H Zola

1. Introduction

Monoclonal antibodies have revolutionized research and diagnosis in medicine and biology. Their impact in treatment of disease has, thus far, been much less impressive than anticipated. There are a number of reasons for the failure of monoclonal antibodies to achieve their perceived potential as therapeutic agents.

One reason is that some of the hoped-for targets simply do not exist. The idea of an antibody-based 'magic bullet' to kill cancer cells presupposes, in its purest form, that cancer cells have on their surface target molecules, which are absent from normal cells. Whilst malignancy is often associated with gene mutations, these do not often code for surface membrane proteins. Nevertheless, antibodies can often kill cancer cells while doing damage to the rest of the body which is real but tolerable.

A second major reason for the relative lack of success of antibodies as therapeutic agents derived from the fact that they are themselves proteins, generally derived from mouse genes, and therefore foreign to the human patient. Patients make an immune response to the mouse protein. At best this limits the effectiveness of second and subsequent doses by clearing the antibody before it can have an effect; at worst hypersensitivity responses to the foreign protein can be life-threatening.

The biological properties of antibody molecules (see *Chapter 1*) lead to additional difficulties in their therapeutic applications. Whole antibody can trigger cells to release factors which initiate inflammation, and the size of the antibody molecule can limit its efficacy, for example by preventing access to solid tumors.

Many of these problems can be solved by engineering the antibody to achieve the desired properties – including size, valency and immunogenicity. This engineering is best done not on the protein but on the gene, because it then needs to be done once only.

Antibody engineering will revolutionize the clinical applications of antibodies, just as Kohler's and Milstein's monoclonal antibody paper revolutionized research and diagnostic aspects of medicine after 1975. The new technologies allow the construction of a wide range of structures (*Figures 3.1* to *3.5*), and phage display and related methods allow the selection of new specificities. Each construct has advantages and disadvantages that allow tailoring properties of engineered antibodies to suit their intended application. The choice of antibody construct to use is an important decision at the beginning of any project involving antigen binding.

2. Choice of antibody designs to suit specific applications

2.1 Overview

The biological properties of antibody constructs are determined by two major features of the molecule. The complementary determining regions (CDR) of the variable Fv-part determine the antigen binding specificity and affinity, whereas additional components such as Fc (in natural immunoglobulin), peptide chains or fusion proteins (in artificial constructs) determine physical properties including stability and solubility, binding valency and effector function.

In artificial constructs, the choice for the Fv-part can either be limited by the specificity of an existing hybridoma cell line or unlimited when phage or ribosomal display is used to screen libraries. The choice for the design of the rest of the molecule is only limited by imagination and technical engineering skills. The choice of construct should be based on biological needs rather than technical possibilities. The smaller an antibody construct is, the better is its tissue penetration and the shorter its serum half-life. In addition, smaller proteins may be less immunogenic.

2.2 Fv antibody fragments

An antibody fragment that retains the correct alignment of the variable light (V_L) chain and variable heavy (V_H) chain also retains the antigen binding specificity and affinity of the parent antibody. The smallest antibody fragments that retain these characteristics are Fv, noncovalently linked heterodimers of V_L and V_H domains with a molecular size of 25 kDa (*Figure 3.1*). Fv-fragments are nonglycosylated and can therefore be produced as functional proteins in bacterial expression systems. However, their assembly in bacteria is often poor, and they readily dissociate into V_L and V_H chains. The Fv molecule can be stabilized by chemical cross-linking, intermolecular disulfide bonding or short peptide linkers between the V_L and V_H domains. The highest stability is achieved by engineering intermolecular disulfide bonds. However, the engineering of disulfide bonds without compromising binding affinity and protein folding requires molecular modelling based on a known three dimensional structure. Engineering of a peptide linker is relatively straightforward, but the effort involved in remodelling the molecule to introduce disulfide bonds may be worthwhile when stability of the Fv fragment is particularly important.

2.3 Single chain Fv (scFv) antibody fragments

V_L and V_H domains joined by a flexible polypeptide linker are transcribed and translated together as a single protein chain, the scFv. The length of the polypeptide linker, its sequence and the order of the domains (V_L-linker-V_H or V_H-linker-V_L) may influence the properties of scFv fragments. Typical linkers consist of repeating sequences of $(Gly_4Ser)_n$. As the distance between the C-terminus of the V_L and the N-terminus of the V_H (39–43 A) is longer

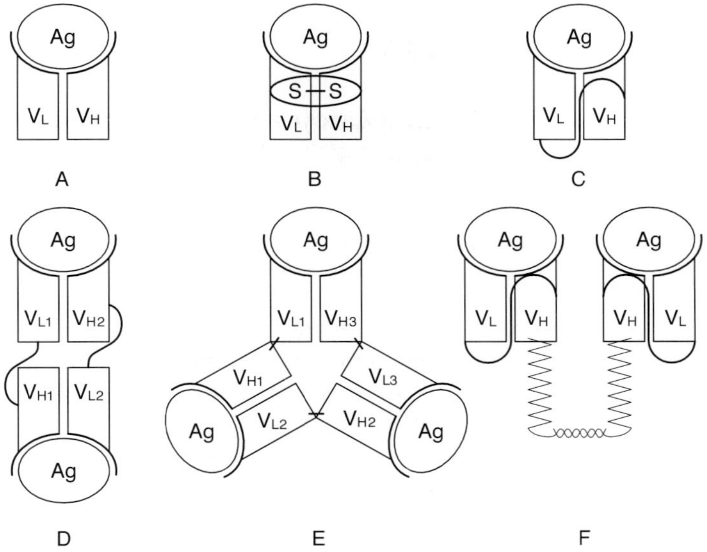

Figure 3.1

Different forms of mono- and multivalent Fv-fragments. (A) nonstabilized Fv-fragment, (B) disulfide stabilized Fv-fragment, (C) single chain Fv-fragment (scFv) – the two domains are stabilized by a short peptide linker, (D) scFv dimer (diabody) that is formed when short peptide linkers are used, (E) scFv trimer that is formed when VL and VH are linked directly, F: two scFv linked by a flexible hinge region.

than the distance between the C-terminus of the V_H and the N-terminus of the V_L (32–34 A) the optimal length is 20–25 amino acids for a VL-linker-V_H and 15–20 amino acids for V_H-linker-V_L fragments (Pluckthun *et al.*, 1996). Shorter linkers (0–10 amino acids) may force the V_L and V_H domain to associate noncovalently with domains of other scFv molecules, resulting in dimers or trimers (*Figure 3.2*).

Linkers as well as the C- or N-terminal ends of V_L and V_H can be designed to incorporate useful features such as diagnostic tags or structures that allow easy radiolabeling or fusion to drugs and toxins. scFv have excellent tissue penetration as compared to Fab fragments or whole antibodies. However, small unbound fragments below the 60 kDa threshold of the glomerular filter undergo rapid renal clearance. Rapid tissue penetration and rapid renal clearance result in a short vascular half-life. This short vascular half-life as well as their small size and lack of glycosylation may explain the low immunogenicity of murine scFv in humans. ScFv lack constant regions and therefore do not activate complement or elicit cytotoxicity.

Probable applications for scFv fragments are in those conditions that require rapid tissue penetration without complement activation and a short intravascular half-life. ScFv fragments are candidates for either topical therapy (taking advantage of rapid penetration) or systemic applications that depend on good tissue penetration and a short half-life, such as radiodiagnostic tumor imaging. However, tumor imaging and therapeutic applications may profit from the extended half-life of Fab fragments,

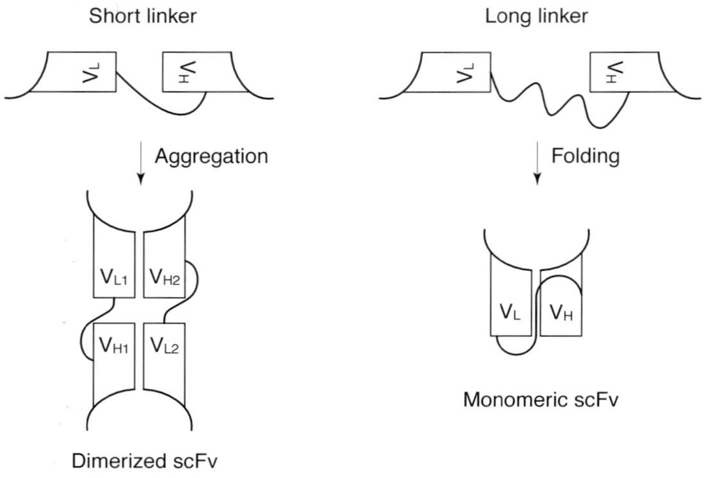

Figure 3.2

Influence of linker length on folding and aggregation. Right: Long peptide linkers (>15 amino acids) are flexible enough to allow the two variable domains to associate to each other without opposing forces. This results in monomeric scFv. Left: Short linkers (<12 amino acids) force the domains to associate with domains from other molecules forming dimers or trimers (domain swapping).

multimeric scFv or fusions of scFv to other proteins and drugs. Depending on the application, scFv can be fused with drugs, enzymes or toxins, incorporated into the surface of immunoliposomes or expressed intracellularly or on the cell membrane.

2.4 Multivalent scFv constructs

Affinity and avidity (sometimes called functional affinity) are important concepts for the discussion of multimeric and multivalent constructs. Affinity is the strength of the binding interaction between a single antigen binding site and an epitope. Affinity depends mostly on the fit between the CDR loops and the epitope of the antigen, and also on additional factors such as temperature and pH. The interaction between the antigen binding site and the epitope of the antigen is a dynamic process with continuous association and dissociation. If a construct has a single antigen-binding site (monovalent construct) the molecule may float freely in solution as soon as its antigen-binding site dissociates from the antigen.

In contrast, a multivalent molecule will bind to two or more epitopes which may be on the same cell membrane or multivalent antigen molecule. If only one binding site dissociates the antibody construct stays in close proximity to the epitope and is likely to reattach to it. Hence, the strength of a multivalent interaction between the antibody construct and the antigen is much higher than the sum of the individual interactions. The strength of multivalent binding is termed avidity, and is illustrated by a dissociation rate 280 times slower for a divalent scFv compared to the monovalent form (Adams *et al.*, 1998).

Avidity depends not only on the antibody valency but also on the density of the antigens on a cell or the multivalency of a soluble antigen. If the distance between two membrane antigens is larger than the maximal distance an antibody can bridge with its binding sites, the binding strength will not be increased by multivalency. On the other hand, if a monovalent antigen is in solution a multivalent antibody fragment may bind several antigens but this will not result in an increase in avidity.

Because of the large gains in binding strength through bivalency much interest has been directed into engineering di- and multivalent antibody fragments. Bivalent scFv have a size and penetration behavior similar to monovalent Fab-fragments, but with increased avidity. With a molecular size of 54–60 kDa dimerized scFv exhibit an extended serum half-life as compared to monovalent scFv fragments due to reduced glomerular filtration.

There are several ways to engineer multivalent scFv-fragments. By reducing the linker length, bivalent scFv can form (*Figure 3.2*). If V_L and V_H are joined directly without a linker, stable trimers with three active antigen-binding sites may be formed (*Figure 3.1*). Another approach is to fuse scFv at the C-terminal end to core-streptavidin, allowing the formation of stable tetrameric complexes. Such constructs can achieve avidity similar to that of whole antibodies. However, the orientation of the binding sites in these multimeric molecules is rigid, in comparison to whole antibodies which have flexible hinge and elbow regions. Multivalent scFv linked by flexible hinge regions, termed miniantibodies, allow bending and rotation (*Figure 3.3*) (Pluckthun and Pack, 1997). Miniantibodies combine the high avidity of whole antibodies with the favorable pharmacokinetics of a small molecule.

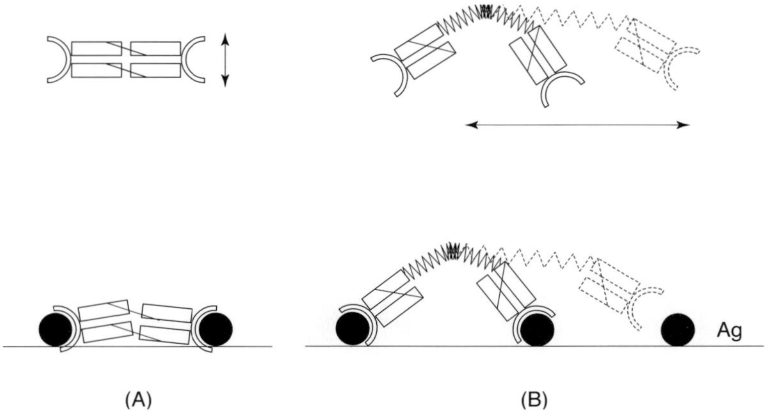

Figure 3.3

Diabodies and miniantibodies (A) Diabodies are formed by domain swapping due to short linker peptides. The two antigen binding sites have a limited flexibility (arrow), allowing multivalent interactions only when antigen density matches the distance between the two antigen binding sites. (B) Miniantibodies are scFv that are linked with highly flexible protein helixes, allowing extensive adaptation to the antigen.

Another interesting variant is the engineering of bispecific molecules with the ability to join two different antigens together. This leads to bispecific but, in regard of each antigen, monovalent molecules. Bispecificity can be achieved with bivalency by engineering bispecific tetramers.

2.5 Fab fragments

Fab fragments consist of a Fv-part plus the light chain constant domain (C_L) and the first heavy constant domain (C_{H1}) (*Figure 3.4*). The extended interface, as compared to Fv-fragments, and the disulfide bond between the constant domains result in excellent stability. Fab show a reduced tissue penetration but extended serum half-life compared with scFv. The prolonged half-life is a disadvantage for *in vivo* diagnostic application but an advantage for therapeutic applications. Murine Fab antibodies are likely to be more immunogenic than scFv, due to the presence of the murine constant region and their longer half-life. Chimeric Fab fragments with human constant regions fused to the murine Fv part can alleviate this problem (*Figure 3.4*).

Fab fragments can be expressed in *E. coli*, but yields of correctly assembled Fab fragments may be lower than for scFv because folding is more complex.

Fab fragments are ideally suited to clinical applications that require an extended intravascular half life without the need for the rapid tissue penetration of scFv or the effector functions of an Fc. An example is the antithrombotic chimeric Fab fragment abciximab (ReoPro) that blocks GPIIb/IIIa receptors on thrombocytes and is widely used clinically with little or no evidence of immunogenicity.

2.6 $F(ab)_2$ fragments

$F(ab)_2$ consist of two Fab-fragments joined by a flexible antibody hinge region (*Figure 3.4*). $F(ab)_2$ fragments can be engineered as monospecific or

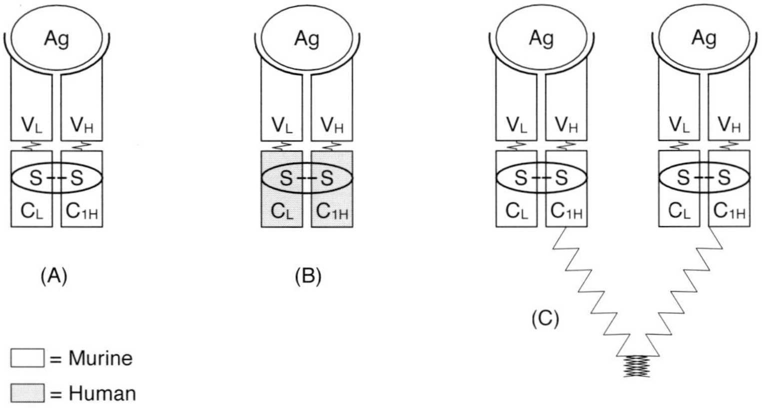

Figure 3.4

Different forms of Fab fragments: (A) murine Fab-fragment, (B) chimeric murine-human Fab-fragment, (C) multivalent F(ab)2-fragments. The two Fab arms are linked with a flexible hinge region, allowing free adaptation to antigen location.

bispecific molecules. Binding properties of monospecific $F(ab)_2$ fragments are similar to those of whole antibodies but they lack the Fc-part that results in complement activation or binding to Fc-receptors on leucocytes.

Typical applications of $F(ab)_2$ fragments include situations where the Fc-part of whole antibody is either not necessary or results in adverse side effects. For example $F(ab)_2$ fragments of CD3 antibody retain full immunosuppressive activity without the lymphokine release syndrome seen with whole antibodies.

Bispecific $F(ab)_2$ fragments can be used to join two cells (e.g. a tumor and a T-cell) to trigger an immune reaction. $F(ab)_2$ fragments have a size of 100 kDa, allowing an extended half life.

Fab and $F(ab)_2$ fragments have been produced for many years by enzymatic digestion of whole antibodies. However, the high costs involved in this procedure have limited their application. Recombinant antibody engineering techniques allow cheap production of these fragments in *E. coli* or other expression systems.

3. Chimeric and humanized whole antibodies

Whole antibodies are required for clinical applications that depend on the long intravascular half-life of these large molecules or the effector function of the Fc-part. However, mouse antibodies recruit human effector function poorly, and repeated injections cause a human antimouse antibody response (HAMA) that results in a decreased half-life and therapeutic effect, and may itself cause disease.

These problems may be alleviated by using chimeric or humanized constructs. Chimeric antibodies are obtained by joining a nonhuman Fv part onto human constant domains (*Figure 3.5*). Engineering of chimeric antibodies is relatively easy and the constructs show identical antigen binding properties to the parent antibodies. Several such constructs have been used successfully in humans with a remarkable reduction in immunogenicity.

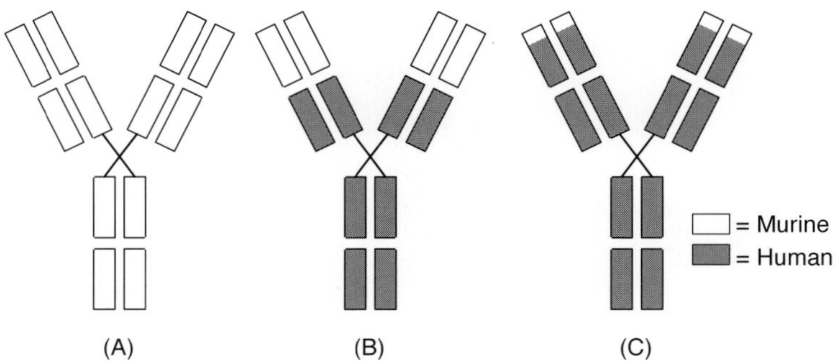

Figure 3.5

Chimeric and humanized whole antibodies: (A) murine antibody, (B) chimeric murine-human antibody; all constant murine domains are replaced by nonimmunogenic human sequences. (C) humanized antibody; only the antigen binding CDR-loops remain murine while all the rest (90%) are human sequences.

A further reduction in immunogenicity may be achieved by humanizing antibodies, by grafting the nonhuman antigen binding loops on to human Fv frameworks (*Figure 3.5*). By this means 90% of the original nonhuman residues are replaced by human structures. This strategy is technically difficult as the conformation of the CDR loops depend on the sequence of the underlying framework. Strategies to improve the CDR conformation include reshaping (in which murine framework sequences are reintroduced at important positions in the human framework to retain the original CDR conformation), or resurfacing (in which a nonhuman Fv domain is humanized by exchanging only those nonhuman framework sequences on the surface of the molecule that come into contact with the immune system).

Humanized antibodies may suffer a loss in binding affinity, requiring remodeling to regain affinity or much higher therapeutic doses to retain efficacy. Further studies on the immunogenicity of humanized antibodies will have to determine whether the increased amount of administered antibody outweighs the reduction in immunogenicity.

Immunogenicity may be avoided by constructing human antibodies directly rather than humanizing murine antibodies. Using phage display it is possible to screen synthetic human libraries for Fab or scFv against the antigen of interest. The use of transgenic mice defective in the production of mouse antibodies but reconstituted with a repertoire of human antibodies provides an approach with enormous potential. Other possible approaches include cloning antibody cDNA from selected lymphocytes or in vitro immunization of human B cells.

An approach for stepwise humanization of murine antibodies is termed 'epitope imprinting' or 'directed selection', where a murine V_H is displayed on phage together with V_L domains amplified from a human library. Selection on antigen binding results in a fragment with a human V_L that pairs the murine V_H. In a second step the human V_L is displayed on phage with a V_H amplified in a human library. The second round of selection results in the final conversion of a murine into a fully human antibody.

4. Single domain antigen binding fragments

The fact that camels possess a class of antibody containing V_H domains without V_L domains has generated some interest in the engineering of single domain antibody fragments. Such fragments, with a molecular size of 12–14 kDa might penetrate tissue barriers even better than Fv fragments, and there are reports of single human V_H domain fragments that exhibit binding specificity and affinity. However, the structural stability of human or murine Fv depends on association between the two domains, and the hydrophobic surface of unmodified V_H and V_L domains limit their solubility when expressed as single domains. The three CDR loops in camel VH domains are longer than the CDR loops in human and murine antibodies and are stabilized by intraloop disulfide bonds. Hence single domain human VH fragments may require additional modification, which may in turn increase immunogenicity.

5. Engineering antibody fragments

5.1 Introduction

The first step in the engineering of any antibody construct is to isolate the V_H and V_L domains. These are subsequently joined together with a peptide linker to form a scFv fragment, or coupled with constant domains to form murine or chimeric Fab- or $F(ab)_2$-fragments. In this section we will focus on the construction of scFv.

5.2 Different strategies to engineer scFv fragments

The genes encoding the V domains can be amplified by polymerase chain reaction (PCR) from hybridomas, blood or tissue lymphocytes or libraries. The easiest way to start is with a hybridoma cell line producing an antibody with the binding specificity of interest. Messenger RNA (mRNA) is reverse transcribed into complementary DNA (cDNA). Hybridomas contain, in addition to the correct mRNA, aberrant mRNA that codes for nonfunctional light and heavy chains, derived from the parent myeloma or spleen cell partner. The total amount of aberrant mRNA may exceed the mRNA of the antibody of interest. One way to isolate the functional sequence is to amplify the V_L and V_H sequences and insert them separately into vectors for bacterial expression. These inserts are then sequenced and compared with known V_L- or V_H-domain sequences (Kabat and Wu, 1991). Sequences which fit with consensus V region genes are then joined together with a linker and the resulting scFv are tested for binding.

Another approach is to neglect the problem of the aberrant chains and join all amplified V_L and V_H products together (Krebber *et al.*, 1997). This leads to a large variety of sequences that are then expressed as scFv proteins, cloned and tested for function. This is done either by picking a number of different clones or by testing large numbers (up to 10^4) of colonies directly on a culture plate. When starting from an immunized animal or library, a much larger number of sequences has to be screened, and this is best done by phage display (see later in this chapter) or ribosomal display panning.

This second approach, as described by Krebber *et al.* (1997) and Pluckthun *et al.* (1996) has proved reliable and easy, allowing successful engineering of scFv fragments often within less than ten days.

The framework regions are well characterized and various sets of degenerate primers for different species have been designed that anneal to sites from which the hypervariable regions can be amplified (Krebber *et al.*, 1997; Pope *et al.*, 1996). The primers can be designed to incorporate fusion tags and the linker sequence.

In a second step the amplified V_L and V_H products are joined together in a splice-overlap-extension (SOE) PCR (*Figure 3.6*) and incorporated into an expression vector. Ten to 50 clones that express protein (detected by slot-blot) are then tested for antigen binding in ELISA or flow cytometry. If this first round of testing is unsuccessful it is necessary to perform large-scale screening by phage display. We have obtained functional scFv from the majority of hybridomas without the need for phage display. Factors which increase the chances of success include the use of mRNA rather than total

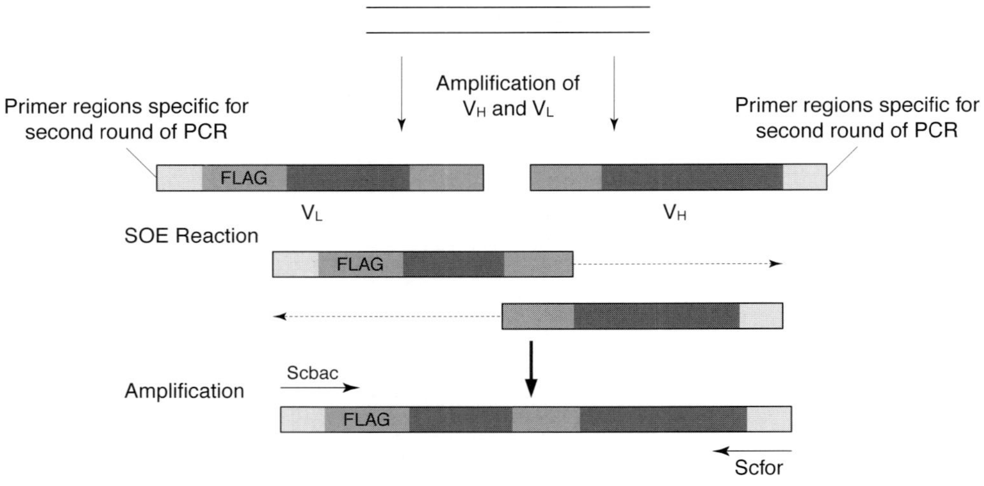

Figure 3.6

Splice overlap extension (SOE) for construction of scFv. The V_H and V_L regions are first amplified from the hybridoma or other source of Ig, using two pairs of primers for the framework 1 and 4 regions of the light and heavy chains. One primer of each pair is modified to code for the linker sequence, while the other member of each pair may be modified to code for a tag (in this case the FLAG peptide), and to include restriction sites for ease of subsequent manipulation. The design of the primers depends on the desired orientation (V_H-V_L or V_L-V_H) of the scFv. V_H and V_L amplifications are done separately; the products are isolated and mixed together. The double-stranded DNA is denatured and allowed to reanneal, at which stage the linker regions hybridize. The polymerase then extends the sequence, forming the spliced product. The two outside primers are now added, and PCR proceeds to amplify the whole product.

RNA, and the quality of the PCR primers. Base deletions within the primers will be amplified into the product and may result in nonfunctional sequences.

5.3 Strategies to improve binding affinity

Generally, high affinity is likely to improve therapeutic efficacy, since a lower concentration will be needed to achieve an equivalent amount of antibody bound to the target. There are exceptions, for example where very high affinity antibody may be 'trapped' by antigen encountered as it penetrates into tissue, and penetration may therefore be inhibited.

Affinity improvement is achieved by mutating the sequence in order to obtain a better fit of the CDR loops to the antigen. Site directed mutagenesis may be used to introduce specific changes based on a known or predicted three dimensional structure of the Fv domains and the antigen. Generally, reliable structural data is lacking, and the preferred approach is affinity maturation by random mutation. This technique introduces a wide variety of random mutations, creating a new 'sublibrary' of sequences including some higher affinity fragments. Mutations are introduced either by taking advantage of the high frequency of errors in the PCR reaction, especially in the presence of manganese, or by using mutator strains of *E. coli*. The mutated sublibrary is then screened by several rounds of panning with phage or ribosomal display, which will select for higher affinity fragments and favor fragments with improved folding properties or with a tendency to dimerize.

6. Expression of antibody fragments

6.1 Overview

Recombinant antibody fragments have been produced in various expression systems such as bacteria, yeast, plants, insect and mammalian cell cultures (Verma *et al.*, 1998). Recombinant antibody fragments can be expressed as correctly folded and directly active proteins or as aggregates requiring *in vitro* refolding to become active. The different expression systems vary in their abilities to fold and secrete recombinant proteins. As a rule, the better the folding abilities of a recombinant protein, the easier and cheaper the necessary expression system. ScFv fragments with good folding properties can be expressed rapidly and at low cost in *E. coli*, while whole antibodies with complicated folding and glycosylation demands require slow and expensive cell culture techniques. The desired antibody format and a suitable expression strategy have to be considered together early in a project. In addition to size, the primary sequence determines folding properties and hence the expression strategy may need to be optimized for each construct. For large-scale production of badly folding proteins it may be necessary to use a more complex expression organism, to re-engineer the recombinant protein, or to apply *in vitro* refolding strategies.

For experimental studies requiring up to 50–100 mg of recombinant protein a stepwise approach to optimizing antibody fragment expression is recommended. In a first step an easy expression system such as *E. coli* should be used. Factors such as enriched culture media, lower expression temperatures, improved aeration and optimized expression vectors may improve expression levels 10- to 100-fold. If these strategies are not successful, it may be necessary to proceed to the second step, a change to a more complex expression organism.

Effector function of whole antibodies depends on glycosylation of the C_{H2} domain, and glycosylation may improve protein solubility. Bacterial expression systems are not able to glycosylate and are therefore not suitable for producing whole antibodies. Yeast, plants, insect and mammalian cell system do glycosylate, although nonhuman glycosylation patterns may result in poor effector function and immunogenicity.

6.2 Antibody fragment expression in *E. coli*

To be functional the antibody fragment molecule must be correctly folded and stabilized by intramolecular disulfide bonds. Both processes take place in the oxidizing environment of the periplasm. Leader sequences such as pelB cause secretion of the translated amino acid chain though the inner cell membrane into the periplasm, where the leader sequence is cleaved off. *E. coli* does not secrete antibody fragments through the outer membrane and hence most functional fragments are found in the periplasmic space. Some protein leaks into the culture medium especially when bacteria start to lyse under suboptimal or extended culture conditions.

Although periplasmic expression of Fab fragments can achieve >95% correctly folded protein, frequently only 1–5% of expressed recombinant protein is correctly folded, the remainder being in an aggregated state as periplasmic or cytoplasmic inclusion bodies, which must be refolded. Refolding may result in yields of up to 40 mg l^{-1} in shake flask cultures and 450 mg l^{-1} in high cell density fermentation. However, refolding requires optimization for each product.

For a simple optimization of recombinant protein production on a small to medium scale, factors such as expression vector, culture media, growth conditions and harvesting strategies have to be optimized. The vector should allow efficient transcription and translation but only in an induced state, as this poses considerable stress on bacteria with the risk of sequence mutation or loss of plasmid (Pluckthun *et al.*, 1996). Culture at 25–27 °C reduces the expression rate and improves folding. A vector with a promoter regulated by a chemical inducer (e.g. lac promotor/lac repressor system) using isopropyl-β-D-galactoside (IPTG) for induction and glucose/lactate for repression, may have an advantage over temperature induced vector systems. Fine tuning of inducer/repressor activity by adding 0–1% glucose controls the expression rate to suit the folding behavior of individual proteins. Expression levels can be further increased with an improved translation initiation sequence (e.g. Shine–Dalgarno SDT7g10).

Other strategies to improve the yield of correctly folded periplasmic protein have focused on coexpression of bacterial proteins that are involved in protein transport and folding. With a range of hybridoma derived scFv, coexpression of the bacterial periplasmic Skp protein (Bothmann and Pluckthun, 1998) improved the yield of correctly folded and soluble periplasmic scFv up to 32-fold in our hands.

Production yields in *E. coli* are often directly proportional to the density of cells in culture. Usually nondefined media such as 2YT or LB are used for small to medium scale expression in shake flasks. These media limit bacterial growth and protein expression as they lack pH buffering. Buffered media such as Terrific Broth (TB) or Super Broth (SB) often allow higher cell densities. Non defined media are rich in nitrogen, but their content of essential elements such as magnesium is unknown. Hence, it is often worthwhile to supplement nondefined media with 5–10 mmol $MgSO_4$ for intact ribosomal activity. In our own experience using TB instead of 2YT medium resulted in 2–3 fold higher yields while a 5 mmol $MgSO_4$ supplement led to better cell viability and reduced loss of recombinant protein into the culture medium. Improved yields of correctly folded and soluble recombinant proteins have been reported for bacterial cultures supplemented with sucrose, glycine/triton X-100 and sorbitol/betaine. However, generalizations are difficult because each construct behaves differently.

Active antibody fragment accumulates mainly in the periplasmic space, which constitutes about 30% of the cell volume and is filled with a peptidoglycan matrix. After vector induction recombinant proteins are expressed during exponential growth phase and possibly to a smaller extent in the first few hours after reaching steady state. Keeping bacteria in culture media for an extended time after optical density at 600 nm (OD_{600}) reaches a plateau (e.g. overnight expression) results in cell lysis and increased leakage into the culture medium.

Antibody fragments can be collected from culture media after centrifugation of cells. This is convenient for small culture volumes, but the concentration of recombinant protein is usually low and unpredictable. Harvesting and purifying antibody fragments from larger cultures is time consuming and cumbersome. ScFv may be precipitated by adding polyethylene glycol 6000 (PEG) or 70% saturated ammonium sulfate. However, this seems to result in low yields and carries the risk of denaturing the proteins.

It is often easier to harvest scFv either as periplasmic or whole cell fraction. This allows the retrieval of recombinant protein in active form at very high concentrations. Whole cell lysate as obtained by a French press or sonication recovers the highest amount of active protein, but this is contaminated with soluble but nonfunctional products. When scFv are intended for administration to animals or humans it is necessary to reduce the amount of contaminating nonfunctional protein. Separation of functional from nonfunctional fragments is difficult, and it is preferable to reduce contamination by recovering soluble proteins from the periplasmic space. Various protocols for recovering periplasmic proteins have been published. A buffer system that uses borate and EDTA (Skerra *et al.*, 1991) retrieves periplasmic proteins effectively, but the periplasm has to be treated repeatedly (up to three times) to obtain most of the protein.

7. Purification of scFv antibody fragments

A variety of different techniques can be used for purification of recombinant antibodies. A popular method utilizes the interaction between a string of five or six histidine residues introduced into the protein and the nickel ion. The recombinant protein can be eluted with imidazole and the resin can be used several times without reconditioning. To obtain very pure protein it may be necessary to combine two different purification systems, for example a nickel column and ion exchange (Pluckthun *et al.*, 1996).

Bacterial endotoxin contamination is a potential problem with antibody fragments expressed in gram negative bacteria. Purification of histidine tagged fragments on nickel columns has been shown to reduce endotoxin contamination (Casey *et al.*, 1995). However, endotoxin binds to histidine at low salt concentration, and therefore buffers with the highest recommended salt concentration should be used. For clinical grade purity it may be necessary to further reduce endotoxin with detoxi gel (Pierce Warriner, Chester, UK) or by the Triton X114 method.

8. Phage display

Phage display is the name given to a technique for the selection of peptides or proteins with binding affinity for a known ligand. In the context of this chapter, the protein being displayed on phage is antibody scFv or Fab, while the ligand is antigen. The defining feature of phage display (and the more recently developed ribosomal display and bacterial display techniques) is that the protein being selected is physically linked to the gene coding its sequence. The consequence of this linkage is that a phage bearing a particular antibody can be selected from a large library of different antibodies by affinity for ligand, and in the same step the gene coding it is isolated.

In phage display this is achieved by inserting the antibody genes linked to the gene for the phage head protein III, which is essential for bacterial infection. Phage display is illustrated diagramatically in *Figures 3.7* and *3.8*.

The application of phage display techniques to antibody fragments has enabled the reproducible production of human monoclonal antibodies (HuMAb). Although an antibody produced by EBV transformed B cells was the first fully human antibody to gain wide approval for clinical use, EBV technology has not been reproducible for cloning of human antibodies. Similarly, transgenic mice are not freely available to researchers for the production of human monoclonal antibodies in mice harboring human antibody repertoires. Furthermore, phage display facilitates *in vitro* affinity maturation and engineering of isotype and structure for unique applications such as bispecific targeting or intracellular immunization.

Phagemid vectors for the surface expression of scFv and Fab on the head of filamentous phage particles are available from a number of commercial or academic sources.

8.1 Practical considerations

There follows a practical discussion of the solid phase selection of combinatorial phage displayed Fab libraries, an *in vitro* correlate of *in vivo* affinity maturation, which is schematically illustrated in *Figure 3.7*.

Vector

Vector choice is prescribed by availability. The generic phagemid vector for directional cloning of Fab libraries and expression of the affinity selected Fab in *E. coli*, is depicted in *Figure 3.8*. Expression of the gene III or cap protein product is important, since it facilitates extrusion of the filamentous phage bearing the Fab fragments on the head of the phage through the *E. coli* periplasmic membrane. The basic elements of the phagemid vector (*Figure 3.8*) are: an effective promoter such as LacZ, a ribosome binding site, a sequence such as pelB to direct the protein to the periplasmic space, a selection marker such as ampicillin resistance and *E. coli* and M13 origins of replication, to allow DNA amplification and phage packaging for panning respectively. Optional extras such as an amber codon between the cap protein (gene III product) and one immunoglobulin chain, to obviate gene III excision, by expression in a suppressor strain of *E. coli*, may be included. Since high copy number is an advantage, many phagemid vectors are based on pUC19 or similar vectors.

Restriction enzyme sites for directional cloning of the heavy chain Fd (V_H-C_{H1}) fragment and light chain should be selected for low frequency of sites in the immunoglobulin database of the species being considered. For example, in the phagemid vector in *Figure 3.8*, the heavy chain Fd fragment is inserted after the light chain, since a considerable number of heavy chains contain SacI and XbaI sites. It should also be noted that approximately 30%

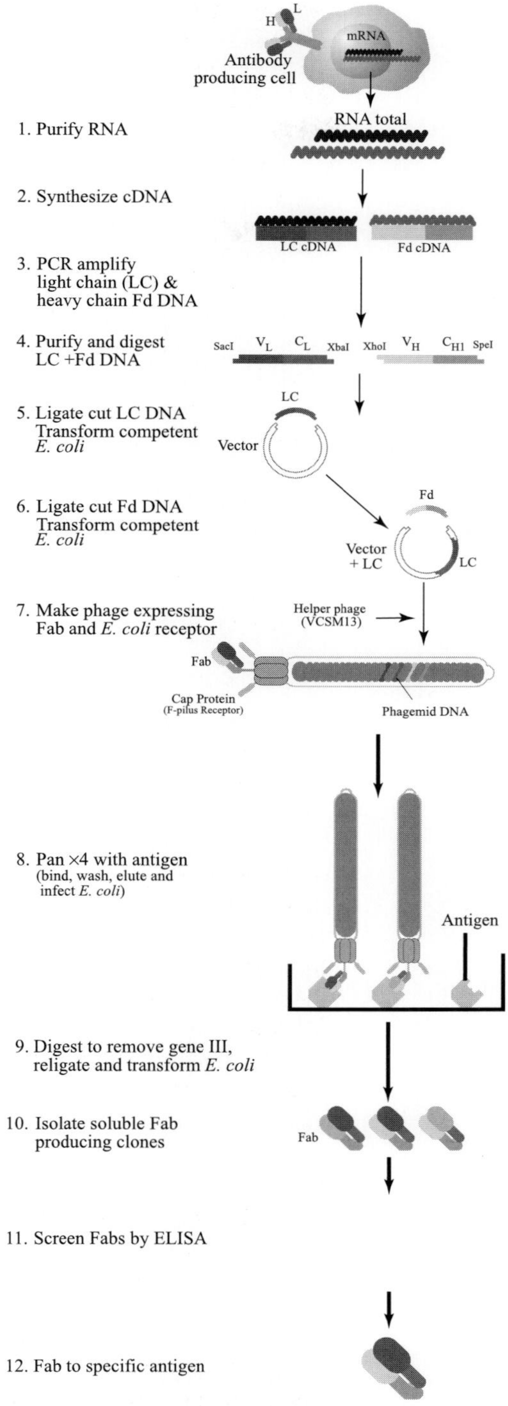

Figure 3.7

Flow diagram of production of and selection of Fab library in phage.

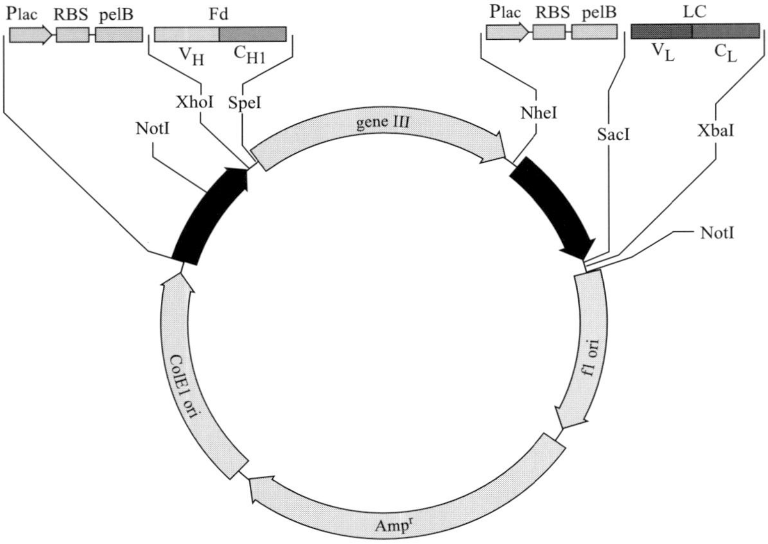

Figure 3.8

Generic phagemid vector for directional cloning of Fab libraries and expression in E. coli.

of human lambda chain genes have SacI sites and therefore when gel purifying digested lambda chain PCR products for insertion into this vector, three major bands are evident. Thirty-three percent of human light chains are lambda chains. Therefore the total proportion of human light chains lost when cloning with this vector is of the order of 10%. However, the presence of an internal enzyme site corresponding to one of the vector cloning sites may be highly relevant, when cloning a single monoclonal antibody via phage display, highlighting the need for sequencing of the antibody prior to cloning.

Antigen

For many pathogens, such as cytomegalovirus (CMV), herpes simplex (HSV) and respiratory syncytial virus (RSV), the antigens and epitopes conferring resistance to the virus are known, and purified, recombinant antigen may be available. The use of pure antigen may facilitate the isolation of antibodies which are clinically relevant, for neutralization of the virus or diagnosis of different strains of the same virus. Cell suspensions, sections and crude lysates have been used successfully to isolate human antibodies by phage display. However it is easier to monitor enrichment of high affinity, antigen specific Fab, when a purified source of antigen is used. In the event that pure antigen is not available, blocking or subtractive panning procedures may be utilized to remove unwanted antibodies. As can be seen in *Table 3.1*, specific Fab enrichment when using a crude antigen can be efficient, in this case achieving a 427-fold increase in relative yield (of eluted to applied phage), from the first to the fifth pan. However, when using unpurified antigen sources, immunodominant antigens may out-

Table 3.1. Panning of a phage displayed human Fab library with virus lysate.

Pan round	Applied phage	Eluted phage	Relative yield
1	1.3×10^{12}	2.8×10^{5}	1.1×10^{-7}
2	5.3×10^{11}	4.7×10^{5}	8.8×10^{-7}
3	1.5×10^{11}	1.4×10^{6}	9.3×10^{-6}
4	3.3×10^{11}	5.8×10^{6}	1.7×10^{-5}
5	1.4×10^{11}	6.7×10^{6}	4.7×10^{-5}

compete the clinically relevant antigen. Conversely the use of highly specific peptides, representing known linear antigenic epitopes, may not always yield high affinity antibodies. More recently, the availability of constrained peptide libraries has introduced a degree of three dimensional structure to the peptides representing antigenic epitopes and this may allow a more comprehensive mimicking of conformation epitopes, in addition to those which are linear in nature.

PCR primer design

For the human and mouse, primers have been designed which include most of the V-region gene families (Larrick *et al.*, 1989; Kang *et al.*, 1991; Marks *et al.*, 1991; Kettleborough *et al.*, 1993; *Table 3.2*). However, it is important to realize the limitations of these primers, which are designed to amplify large libraries. When amplifying an individual antibody from a hybridoma or EBV transformed cell line, it is an advantage to know the sequence of the antibody in order to optimize the primer choice. Some measure of the diversity of antibodies amplified may be obtained by the number of different clones isolated, after panning or selection of the libraries, with several antigens. This type of analysis should be a more statistically efficient means of sampling library diversity than DNA sequencing of random clones. As an alternative measure of diversity and primer efficiency, the library should include a representation of all heavy chain and light chain v-region gene families in the antigen selected clones. However one must keep in mind the high proportional representation of some gene families such as V_{H3} and V_{K3}.

Library size: immune vs naive and memory

The percentage of clones with both heavy chain Fd and light chain inserts also determines library size, as a library of 10^8 clones with only 10% double inserts effectively contains only 10^7 clones. The percentage of clones bearing both inserts is determined by DNA restriction enzyme digestion. It is probably not necessary to utilize large libraries of 10^9 to 10^{11} clones when immune donors are used as the library source, because there will be an enrichment of clones specific for the antigen of interest. Furthermore, immune donors are a source of *in vivo* affinity matured antibodies, which in many cases have also been selected for functional activity (e.g. pathogen neutralization) *in vivo*.

Memory B-cells may be cloned from the bone marrow even when no antibody is found in peripheral blood. The repertoire of circulating blood cells is more limited, representing mostly current or recent antibody responses.

***Table* 3.2.** Human immunoglobulin heavy chain Fd primers

Heavy chain V-region 5′ primers		
V_{H13a}	5′ – AG GTG CAG CTC GAG (C/G)AG TCT GGG – 3′	(23 mer)
V_{H134f}	5′ – AG GTG CAG CTG CTC GAG TC(T/G) GG – 3′	(22 mer)
V_{H2f4g}	5′ – CAG GTG CAG CTA CTC GAG T(C/G)G GG – 3′	(23 mer)
V_{H6a}	5′ – CAG GTA CAG CTC GAG CAG TCA GG – 3′	(23 mer)
Fd 3′ primers (Kang et al., *1991)*		
IgG1		
CG1z	5′ – GCA TGT ACT AGT TTT GTC ACA AGA TTT GGG – 3′	(30 mer)
IgG2		
CG2a	5′ – CTC GAC ACT AGT TTT GCG CTC AAC TGT CTT – 3′	(30 mer)
IgG3		
CG3a	5′ – TGT GTG ACT AGT GTC ACC AAG TGG GGT TTT – 3′	(30 mer)
IgG4		
CG4a	5′ – GCA TGA ACT AGT TGG GGG ACC ATA TTT GGA – 3′	(30 mer)
IgM		
CM1	5′ – GCT CAC ACT AGT AGG CAG CTC AGC AAT CAC – 3′	(30 mer)
IgD		
CD1	5′ – TGC CTT ACT AGT CTC TGG CCA GCG GAA GAT – 3′	(30 mer)
IgE		
CE1	5′ – GCT GAA ACT AGT GTT GTC GAC CCA GTC TGT GGA – 3′	(33 mer)
IgA		
CA1	5′ – AGT TGA ACT AGT TGG GCA GGG CAC AGT CAC – 3′	(30 mer)
Human light chain primers		
Kappa chain V-region 5′ primers		
V_{K14}	5′ – GAC ATC GAG CTC ACC CAG TCT CC – 3′	(23 mer)
V_{K2a}	5′ – GAT ATT GAG CTC ACT CAG TCT CCA – 3′ (Kang *et al.*, 1991)	(24 mer)
V_{K3b}	5′ – GAA ATT GAG CTC AC(G/A) CAG TCT CCA – 3′	(24 mer)
Lambda chain V-region 5′ primers		
V_{L1gp}	5′ – AAT TTT GAG CTC ACT CAG CCC CCC TCT GTG TC	(29 mer)
V_{L2-4}	5′ – TCT GHV GAG CTC CAG SMB SCY KYH GTG TCT GTG – 3′	(30 mer)
V_{L5-8}	5′ – CAG DCT GAG CTC ACG CAG SMG YCY TCC – 3′	(27 mer)
Constant region 3′ primers (Kang et al., *1991)*		
Kappa		
CK1d	5′ – GCG CCG TCT AGA ATT AAC ACT CTC CCC TGT TGA AGC TCT TTG TGA CGG GCG AAC TCA G – 3′	(57 mer)
Lambda		
CL2	5′ – CGC CGT CTA GAA CTA TGA ACA TTC TGT AGG – 3′	(30 mer)

Factors affecting efficiency of transformation and library size

The efficiency of transformation of the host *E. coli* depends on several factors. Efficiency of the ligation reaction is a major factor, in turn affected by age and heat stability (at room temperature) of the ligase enzyme or inactivation of the ligase by residual alcohol from precipitation, residual glass beads from purification, or residual agarose if ligation certified agarose is not used. High salt concentrations in the ligated vector DNA can cause arcing in the electroporation procedure. Therefore ethanol precipitation of ligated DNA and dissolving in nuclease free water, prior to electroporation, is advised. Other methods of transformation, such as the use of calcium, are not efficient enough for the library sizes usually required for phage display. Other factors of major importance for electroporation efficiency are the total amount of DNA and the electrocompetence of the *E. coli*, which can be measured with a standard vector such as pUC19.

Assuming the electrocompetence of the *E. coli* is 10^9 μg^{-1} of pUC19 DNA, freshly ligated phagemid DNA such as that of the vector depicted in *Figure 3.8* will be about 100-fold less efficient. Any further sub optimal conditions will reduce the transformation efficiency and library size correspondingly. If a library size greater than 10^7 μg^{-1} is needed, *E. coli* of greater electrocompetence than 10^9 μg^{-1} must be used. *E. coli* of 10^9 μg^{-1} to 5×10^9 μg^{-1} competence is available commercially. With extreme attention to removal of salt by extensive washing in 10% glycerol, minimization of processing time and temperature (processing on ice, in a cold room), electrocompetence of 10^{10} μg^{-1} to 10^{11} μg^{-1} DNA can be achieved. The amount of DNA used for the transformation is also important. Usually for a vector such as that depicted in *Figure 3.8*, 2.5 to 10 μg^{-1} is optimal. At DNA levels 10-fold higher, lower transformation efficiencies may be seen.

Solid phase selection and affinity

Solid phase selection procedures such as panning select phage on the basis of affinity. Increases in relative yield (*Table 3.1*) of the order of 100-fold to 1000-fold are usually sufficient to isolate Fab clones of 10^{-11}M affinity. Acid elution is generally the most practical means of phage recovery, although antigen or existing antibodies may also be used.

Screening of Fab clones

When screening Fab clones for activity and specificity, it is important to be aware of the law of mass action. Individual Fab clones may produce from micrograms to milligrams protein per liter. This >1000-fold range in antibody concentration may confound interpretation, with some Fab clones appearing specific due to low protein concentration and others appearing nonspecific due to high concentration. Clones should be purified and titrated at appropriate protein concentrations (i.e. between μg ml^{-1} and pg ml^{-1}), with both the selection antigen and an unrelated antigen. In the case of a recombinant antigen with attached fusion protein, the best negative control antigen may be the fusion protein. A different viral antigen or a similar protein of a distantly related virus may be appropriate for some viral antigens. For crude virus lysates, a lysate prepared from uninfected cells may be used as a negative control. Similarly for lysates of malignant cells an autologous, nonmalignant cell type (e.g. fibroblasts or lymphocytes) is optimal. In most cases the antigen used for blocking, often bovine serum albumin or powdered milk, is a good antigen for screening out polyreactive antibodies.

Protein yield in *E. coli* is not necessarily important, depending on the final antibody application. If the Fab requires engineering into a whole antibody molecule, the eventual expression system will most likely be mammalian, yeast or plant and yields in these systems will bear no relation to those in *E. coli*. What is important is that enough Fab can be purified for characterization. Usually 100 mg of purified Fab is sufficient for preliminary characterization, including some functional testing. Purification of Fab is necessary for most functional testing, due to the inhibitory effects of endotoxins and other contaminating molecules.

Detection or purification of antibody fragments may be via a peptide or protein fused to the fragment or via antihuman Fab/Fv fragment antibodies. *Figure 3.9* demonstrates the 99.9% purity achievable using a highly specific antihuman Fab linked to agarose beads. However in some cases it may be

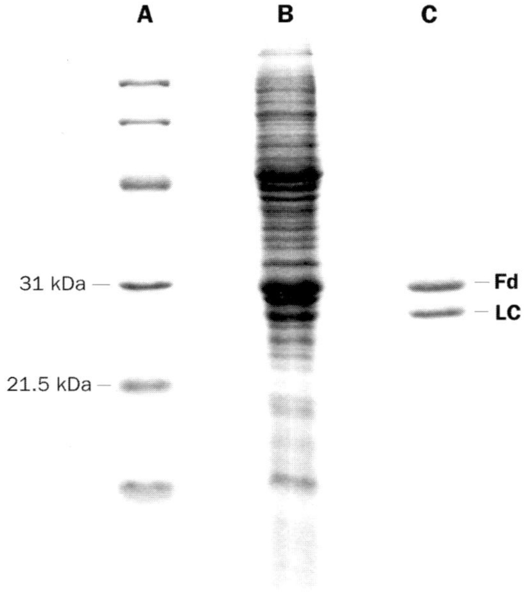

Figure 3.9

Purification of recombinant human Fab to respiratory syncytial virus (RSVF2-5) from E. coli *strain XL1-Blue periplasmic extract, by affinity chromatography, using goat antihuman Fab (Bethyl Laboratories, Montgomery, TX) linked to CNBr activated Sepharose 4B (Pharmacia). SDS-PAGE (4/15% gel) analysis of* E. coli *extract post-induction with IPTG and affinity purified Fab. Lane A, molecular weight markers; lane B,* E. coli *cell extract (5μg of protein, representing 1% of total Fab from the periplasmic extract obtained by freeze/thawing three times in 25 ml PBS/0.01% NaN_3/0.2mM PMSF, was boiled in sample buffer); lane C, RSVF2-5 Fab concentrated from affinity column eluate after loading, washing with 1 l of PBS, eluting in 50 ml 0.2 M glycine (pH 2.5) and neutralizing with 5 ml 1 M Tris (pH 9).*

necessary to have a peptide or protein tag on the Fab, particularly when the target tissue expresses immunoglobulin. It may be more practical to screen by detecting phage directly, using commercial anti-M13 antibodies.

The choice of screening method may vary depending on the intended application of the antibody. It is relatively simple to screen hundreds of clones by ELISA. Immunohistochemical or flow cytometry screening are more laborious and it may be more practical to perform a preliminary screen by ELISA. However, in our experience, only 20% of high affinity Fab or scFv isolated using ELISA screening with recombinant antigen show cell binding by flow cytometry or immunohistochemistry.

8.2 Engineering for functional activity or higher affinity

Antibodies isolated by screening libraries may be of low affinity, polyreactive, or nonfunctional (e.g. non neutralizing for the intended pathogen). An antibody of affinity less than 10^{-8} M is effectively non-functional both *in vitro* and *in vivo*. In this situation phage display provides a rapid approach to engineering new antibodies with altered specificity and affinity (see *Section 5.3*).

Further reading

McCafferty, J., Hoogenboom, H. and Chiswell, D. (eds) (1996) *Antibody Engineering: A Practical Approach*. Oxford University Press, Oxford.

References

Adams, G.P., Schier, R., McCall, A.M., Crawford, R.S., Wolf, E.J., Weiner, L.M. and Marks J.D. (1998) Prolonged *in vivo* tumour retention of a human diabody targeting the extracellular domain of human HER2/neu. *Br. J. Cancer* **77**, 1405–1412.

Bothmann, H. and Pluckthun, A. (1998) Selection for a periplasmic factor improving phage display and functional periplasmic expression. *Nature Biotechnol.* **16**, 376–380.

Casey, J.L., Keep, P.A., Chester, K.A., Robson, L., Hawkins, R.E. and Begent R.H. (1995) Purification of bacterially expressed single chain Fv antibodies for clinical applications using metal chelate chromatography. *J. Immunol. Methods* **179**, 105–116.

Kabat, E.A. and Wu, T.T. (1991) Identical V region amino acid sequences and segments of sequences in antibodies of different specificities. Relative contributions of VH and VL genes, minigenes, and complementarity-determining regions to binding of antibody-combining sites. *J. Immunol.* **147**, 1709–1719.

Kang, A.S., Burton, D.R. and Lerner, R.A. (1991) Combinatorial immunoglobulin libraries in phage lambda. In: *Methods: A Companion to Methods in Enzymology*, vol. 2, p.111 (Lerner, R.A. and Burton, D.R. eds). Academic Press.

Kettleborough, C.A., Saldanha, J., Ansell, K.H. and Bendig, M.M. (1993) Optimisation of primers for cloning libraries of mouse immunoglobulin genes using PCR. *Eur. J. Immunol.* **23**, 206–211.

Krebber, A., Bornhauser, S., Burmester, J., Honegger, A., Willuda, J., Bosshard, H.R. and Plückthun A. (1997) Reliable cloning of functional antibody variable domains from hybridomas and spleen cell repertoires employing a reengineered phage display system. *J. Immunol. Methods* **201**, 35–55.

Larrick, J.W., Danielson, L., Brenner, C.A., Wallace, E.F., Abrahamson, M., Fry, K.E. and Borrebaek C.A.K. (1989) Polymerase chain reaction using mixed primers:

Cloning of human monoclonal antibody variable region genes from single hybridoma cells. *Bio/Technology* **7** 934–938.

Marks, J.D., Tristrem, M., Karpas, A. and Winter, G. (1991) Oligonucleotide primers for polymerase chain reaction amplification of human immunoglobulin variable genes and design of family-specific oligonucleotide probes. *Eur. J. Immunol.* **21**, 985–991.

Persson, M., Caothien, R.H. and Burton, D.R. (1991) Generation of diverse high-affinity human monoclonal antibodies by repertoire cloning. *Proc. Natl Acad. Sci. USA* **88**, 2432–2436.

Plückthun, A. and Pack, P. (1997). New protein engineering approaches to multivalent and bispecific antibody fragments. *Immunotechnology* **3**, 83–105.18.

Plückthun, A., Krebber, A., Krebber, C., Horn, U., Knüpfer, U., Wenderoth, R., Nieba, L., Proba, K. and Riesenberget, D. (1996) Producing antibodies in *Escherichia coli*: from PCR to fermentation. In: *Antibody Engineering: A Practical Approach*, pp. 203–252 (McCafferty, J., Hoogenboom, H., Chiswell, D. eds). Oxford University Press, Oxford.

Pope, A., Embleton, M. and Mernaugh, R. (1996) Construction and use of antibody gene repertoires. In: *Antibody Engineering: A Practical Approach*, pp. 1–40 (McCafferty, J., Hoogenboom, H., Chiswell, D. eds). Oxford University Press, Oxford.

Skerra, A., Pfitzinger, I. and Pluckthun, A. (1991) The functional expression of antibody Fv fragments in *Escherichia coli*: improved vectors and a generally applicable purification technique. *Biotechnology* **9**, 273–278.

Verma, R., Boleti, E. and George, A.J.T. (1998) Antibody engineering: Comparison of bacterial, yeast, insect and mammalian expression systems. *J. Immunol. Methods* **216**, 165–181

Protocol 3.1

Preparation and selection of phage display library of Fab fragments

Solutions, buffers and media

Use MilliQ or equivalent water throughout

10 × PBS 2 l: 174 g NaCl, 21g Na_2HPO_4, 7.7g NaH_2PO_4, add H_2O to 2 l and stir until dissolved. Store at room temp

PBS/0.05% Tween 20 l: 2 l PBS 10 ×, 10 ml Tween, add H_2O to 20 l, mix and store at room temp

ELISA (alkaline phosphatase) diluent 1 l: 2.03 g $MgCl_2.6H_2O$, 8.4 g Na_2CO_3, 1.0 g NaN_3 (toxic, wear gloves and mask). Make up to 950 ml with H_2O, adjust to pH 9.8, make up to 1 l and autoclave

Elution buffer (Panning) 200 ml: 1.6 ml 12 M HCl, 150 ml H_2O, adjust to pH 2.2 with solid glycine, make up to 200 ml with H_2O, check pH. Autoclave (or add 0.2 g BSA and filter, for synthetic libraries)

2% agarose (for DNA 70–1000 bp) 200 ml: To a 500 ml bottle add 1 × TAE 200 ml, 2 g UltraPure agarose (Gibco BRL #5510UA), 2 g NuSeive GTG agarose (low melting point, Cat. # 50082); microwave on full power for 3 min, cool to room temperature before storing or add 20 μl of 10 mg ml^{-1} EtBr and pour gel for electrophoresis

0.6% agarose (for DNA 300–10 000 bp) 200 ml: To a 500 ml bottle add 1 × TAE 200 ml, 1.2 g UltraPure agarose and proceed as for 2% agarose

LB agar: 32 g l^{-1} in H_2O; autoclave then dispense 250 ml aliquots into sterile 500 ml bottles. Store at 4°C

LB broth: 20 g l^{-1} in H_2O, then as for LB agar

Tetracyline stock (5 mg ml^{-1}) 50 ml: 250 mg in 50 ml EtOH, filter through 0.2 μm membrane and dispense 1.0 ml into sterile 1.5 ml 'microfuge tubes'. Store at –20°C

Carbenicillin stock (100 mg ml^{-1}) 100 ml: Dissolve 10 g carbenicillin in 100 ml H_2O, filter through 0.2 μm membrane and dispense 1.0 ml into sterile 1.5 ml 'microfuge tubes'. Store at –20°C

0.1M bicarbonate buffer pH 8.6 (Antigen binding) 1 l: 8.4 g $NaHCO_3$ l^{-1} H_2O. Adjust pH to 8.6, filter through 0.2 μm membrane and store at 4°C

SOC (= SOB + Glucose + $MgCl_2$): First make up SOB 1 l: Bacto tryptone 20 g, Bacto yeast extract 5 g, NaCl 0.5 g. Dissolve in 950 ml H_2O and add 10 ml 25 nM KCl (1.86 g/100 ml). Adjust pH to 7.0 with 5 M NaOH. Adjust to 1 l and autoclave in 100 ml aliquots (or filter if urgent). Store at room temp. To make up SOC: 100 ml SOB, add 2 ml sterile filtered 2 M glucose (18 g/100 ml) and 5 ml 2 M $MgCl_2$ (sterilized by autoclaving)

6 × load buffer 100 ml: 0.25 g bromophenol blue, 40 g sucrose, make up to 100 ml in H_2O. Store at 4°C

EtBr plates (for determination of DNA concentration): 0.6 g agarose, make up to 100 ml in TAE and microwave at full power for 3 min. Cool until possible to hold bottle, add 10 μl EtBr (10 mg ml^{-1}). Pour 20 ml per Petri dish

Top agar: 1 g bacto tryptone, 0.5 g NaCl, 0.65 g agar (Difco 0138-05-0), add 100 ml H_2O. Autoclave. Remelt in microwave, use at 45°C.

Alternatively dilute LB agar: LB broth at 1:1, microwave and use at 45°C

Super broth (SB): 30 g Bacto tryptone, 20 g Bacto yeast extract, 10 g MOPS (3-(N-morpholine)-propane-sulfonic acid); add H_2O to 1 l and adjust pH to 7.0. Autoclave.

Carbenicillin plates: Add 16 g LB agar to 500 ml H_2O in a 1 l bottle. Autoclave then add 25 ml 2 M glucose. Add 500 μl of carbenicillin stock (100 mg ml^{-1}) immediately before pouring plates

Tetracycline plates: Add 16 g LB agar to 500 ml H_2O in a 1 l bottle. Autoclave, then add 25 ml 2 M glucose. Add 1 ml of tetracycline stock (5 mg ml^{-1}) immediately before pouring plates.

Tris EDTA (TE): 1 M Tris.HCl 10 ml, EDTA 1 mM (0.372 g), make up to 1 l with H_2O and adjust pH to 7.4; autoclave

Protocol Part A – Preparation of electrocompetent E. coli *XL1-blue*

1. Inoculate 10 μl from a frozen stock, or a single colony from an overnight plate culture (tetracycline (Tet) 10 μg ml^{-1}), into 10 ml of Superbroth (SB) (Tet 10 μg ml^{-1}).
2. Incubate on a shaker (~ 200 rpm) overnight at 37°C.
3. Inoculate 1 ml of this overnight culture into 1 l of SB with 10 ml of 2 M glucose added (no Tet) first thing in the morning.
4. Incubate for ~5 h at 37°C on a shaker until the OD_{600} = 1.0.
5. Chill (4°C) culture for 15–30 min, centrifuge at 1500 **g** for 20 min at 4°C.
6. Wash 3 × with cold (4°C), sterile H_2O /10% glycerol, in decreasing volumes of 500 ml, 250 ml, and 120 ml, centrifuging as above.
7. Resuspend cells to a total volume of 3 ml in 10% glycerol in sterile H_2O.
8. Aliquot 200 μl or 40 μl volumes into tubes in an ethanol/dry ice bath so that they freeze immediately.
9. Store at –80 to –70°C.
10. To test competence mix 0.1 ng pUC19 with 40 μl of the freshly thawed XL1-Blue and pulse at 1.25 kV (0.1 cm gap cuvette), flush cuvette with 3 ml SOC and incubate transformed cells for 1 h at 37°C, dilute with 10 ml SB and plate 100, 10, and 1 μl volumes on LB/carb plates. Efficiency should be >10^9 transformants/μg pUC19.

Notes

Steps 1–7 are performed on ice and all washing is performed in the cold room.

Instead of preparing electrocompetent *E. coli*, they may be purchased from Stratagene (La Jolla, CA) or Life Technologies (Grand Island, NY).

Protocol Part B – M13 helper phage preparation

1. Inoculate 2 x 15 μl frozen/thawed *E. coli* XL1-Blue into 2 × 100 ml prewarmed (37°C) SB with tetracycline (10 μg ml^{-1}) and incubate at 37°C for 2 h or until the culture reaches OD_{600} ~ 0.5.
2. Add 50 μl of VCSM13 helper phage supernatant containing 10^{12} pfu/ml (or equivalent amount of VCSM13) to each 100 ml culture.
3. Incubate at 37°C for 1 h on a shaker (200 rpm).
4. Add kanamycin to 70 μg ml^{-1} and incubate for a further 3–4 h at 37°C.
5. Centrifuge at 2500 **g** for 15 min.
6. Incubate supernatant for 20 min at 70°C then recentrifuge as above.
7. Store as 50 ml volumes at 4°C.
8. Titrate on prewarmed agar plates with no antibiotics as follows:
   (a) Melt top agar and cool to 42°C.
   (b) Aliquot *E. coli* XL1-Blue in 100 μl volumes (from a fresh culture at OD_{600} = 1).
   (c) Make serial dilutions of the VCSM13 helper phage (10^{-6}, 10^{-8}, 10^{-10}, 10^{-12}) in LB broth.
   (d) Add 1 μl of each dilution to 100 μl of XL1-Blue; add this to 3 ml of top agar and pour onto a dry, warm (37°C) base agar plate (without antibiotics).
   (e) Incubate overnight at 37°C and count plaques the following day.
9. Aliquot the helper phage at 10^{12} pfu/vial and store at 4°C for use.

Notes

Each dilution should be made with a fresh tip. All dilutions (i.e. including the initial 10 μl/1 ml) should be made in LB broth.

After two amplifications from phage stocks it is necessary to isolate a single plaque and amplify fresh helper phage, to obviate accumulation of deletions.

Protocol Part C – Isolation of RNA

Suitable material encoding the Fd and kappa or lambda light chains may be prepared using a standard guanidine isothiocyanate RNA extraction (e.g. Stratagene, Cat. # 200344). For the synthesis of cDNA, either mRNA or total RNA may be used. The starting point is human lymphocytes or plasma cells (10^7–10^8 total), purified from blood, marrow or lymphoid tissue by standard methods. Volumes below are given for 5 × 10^6 lymphocytes.

1. Prepare denaturant guanidine isothiocyanate (solution D) by adding 7.2 ml β-mercaptoethanol per ml of denaturing solution.
2. Add 0.5 ml of solution D per 5 × 10^6 lymphocytes to the cell pellet, resuspend the cell pellet and transfer to a sterile 1.5 ml microcentrifuge tube (0.5 ml per tube).
3. Add 0.05 ml of 2 M sodium acetate, pH 4. Mix by inversion.
4. Add 0.5 ml of phenol saturated with water. Mix by inversion.
5. Add 0.1 ml of chloroform:isoamyl alcohol mixture. Vortex or shake vigorously for 10 s and chill on ice for 15 min. If two layers do not form add another volume of chloroform:isoamyl alcohol and repeat.
6. Centrifuge in a microcentrifuge at 14 000 rpm for at least 15 min at 4°C.
7. Transfer the upper aqueous phase to a fresh tube, add an equal volume of isopropanol, 1 μl of glycogen and store for 1 h at –20°C to precipitate RNA.

   The sample may be shipped, preferably on dry ice, at this stage.
8. Centrifuge at 14 000 **g** as above, for at least 15 min at 4°C to pellet RNA.
9. Resuspend the pellets from each microcentrifuge tube in 0.5 ml of solution D.
10. Add 0.5 ml of isopropanol, mix well and store at –20°C for cDNA preparation by reverse transcriptase (RT).
11. Pellet the RNA at 14 000 rpm in a microcentrifuge for 15 min.
12. Wash the RNA pellet in 1 ml 75% ethanol/DEPC treated water (or other nuclease free water) and recentrifuge as step 11.
13. Dry carefully at room temperature or under vacuum for ~5 min so as not to dry the RNA pellet completely.
14. Dissolve the RNA in 25 μl of DEPC treated (or nuclease free) water and remove an aliquot (2–5 μl) to determine absorbance at 260 and 280 nm.
15. Determine the RNA purity and concentration:

    Absorbance 260/Absorbance 280 should be >2.0 (lower values indicate protein and/or phenol contamination).

    RNA concentration (μg ml^{-1}) = Absorbance at 260 nm x dilution factor x 40

Notes

An immunized mouse would normally generate 5–10 μg RNA μl^{-1} from a spleen.

Human peripheral blood or bone marrow lymphocytes would normally yield 1–5 μg μl^{-1} from 50 ml and 5 ml respectively.

Protocol Part D – Generation of cDNA by reverse transcriptase (RT)

1. Add 10–30 μg of total RNA to a sterile 1.5 ml microcentrifuge tube.
2. Add 3 μl (60 pmoles) of heavy or light chain 3′ primer or 2 μl (1 μg) oligodT then make up to 27 μl with nuclease free or DEPC treated water.

3. Heat at 70°C for 10 min then cool to 4°C.
4. Add 2 μl RNAse inhibitor (e.g. RNAsin, Promega, 40 u μl^{-1}).
5. Add 10 μl 5 × RT buffer.
6. Add 3 μl dNTPs (25 mM each of dATP, dCTP, dGTP, dTTP) (e.g. Ultrapure dNTP kit, Pharmacia).
7. Add 5 μl of 0.1 M DTT.
8. Make up to 48 μl using DEPC water before adding enzyme.
9. Add 2 μl (200 u) reverse transcriptase (e.g. Life Technologies Superscript RT).
10. Incubate at room temp. for 10 min, then 42°C for 50 min.
11. Terminate reaction by incubating at 90°C for 5 min, then at 4°C for 10 min.
12. Add 1 μl (1 u μl^{-1}) of RNAse H and incubate at 37°C for 20 min.

Protocol Part E – PCR amplification of Fd and light chains

1. Add 90 μl of freshly prepared PCR mix (792 μl DNase free water + 100 μl 10 × Taq buffer + 8 μl dNTPs (dATP, dCTP, dGTP, and dTTP each at 25 mM) to each PCR reaction tube.
2. Add 3 μl of 5′ and 3 μl of 3′ primers, 60 pmoles of each (i.e. each at 20 μM).
3. Add 0.5 μl (5 units) of Taq polymerase (Promega, Perkin Elmer etc.).
4. Add 2 μl of cDNA (originally containing ~ 2 μl of RNA).
5. Add two drops of mineral oil and carry out 25–40 rounds of PCR amplification.
6. For the Perkin Elmer 9600: 94°C for 15 s
   52°C for 50 s
   72°C for 1.5 min
   followed by a final incubation at 72°C for 10 min.
   For old 'Thermal cyclers" replace above times with: 1 min, 1 min, 3 min.
7. Remove 10 μl of PCR reaction product, add 2 μl of 6 × load buffer and run on a 2% agarose gel (50:50 of normal:low melting-point agarose) with Phi 174/Hae III marker.
8. A strong band about 660 bp should be indicative of successful PCR amplification of DNA encoding the Fd (V_H + C_{H1} regions) or light chain (V_L + C_L regions).

Protocol Part F – PCR product quantification

1. Pool PCR products with common 3′ primers i.e., Fds or kappa or lambda light chains.
2. Extract twice with an equal volume of phenol/chloroform.
3. Add 1/10 vol. of 3 M sodium acetate pH 5.2 and 2 vol. of ethanol and incubate at –20°C overnight (alternatively add 3 vol. of ethanol and incubate at –70°C for 1–2 h).

4. Centrifuge at 10 000 **g** in a microcentrifuge for 15 min at 4°C, to obtain DNA pellet.
5. Add 0.2 ml of 70% ethanol, rinse the tube and discard the liquid.
6. Dry the pellet under vacuum for 5 min (or air dry).
7. Resuspend DNA in 50 μl of TE. Determine absorbance at 260 nm and 280 nm to quantify DNA in sample and check DNA concentration by EtBr plate.
8. Add 10 μl of 6 × load buffer and run on a 2% agarose gel (50:50 of normal:low melting-point agarose) with Phi 174/Hae III marker.
9. Cut out the bands at 639–699 bp (i.e. light chain or Fd DNA) from the gel and recover by Qiaex (Qiagen), electroelution (Elutrap, Schleicher and Schuell) or other method.
10. Determine the concentration of DNA for digestion with XhoI/SpeI (Fd) or SacI/XbaI (light chain) for ligation into the vector.

Protocol Part G – Restriction enzyme digestion of PCR products (Fd or light chain) for ligation into the vector (Tables 3.3 and 3.4)

1. Digest ~2 mg of pooled Fd with one equivalent each of XhoI (140 u) and SpeI (34 u) with 10 ml 10 × buffer (buffer 2, New England Biolabs; buffer H, Boehringer-Mannheim), in a total volume of 100 μl (make up to 100 μl with nuclease free water), for 3 h at 37°C.
2. Digest ~2 mg of pooled light chain (LC) DNA with one equivalent each of SacI (70 u) and XbaI (140 u) with 10 μl 10 × buffer (buffer 4, New England Biolabs; buffer A, Boehringer-Mannheim), in a total volume of 100 μl (make up to 100 μl with nuclease free water), for 3 h at 37°C.
3. Gel purify each digest in 2% agarose as above for ligation into digested vector, vector + Fd (for ligation of cut light chain DNA) or vector + LC (for ligation of cut Fd DNA), as above.
4. Ligate cut, gel purified vector, vector + Fd or vector + LC as from steps 17. or 24. 'H. Vector Preparation.'

Table 3.3. Equivalent enzyme amounts for cutting vector and PCR inserts (3 h, 37°C):

	Vector (1mg)	**PCR inserts (1mg)**
NheI	10 u	
SpeI	3 u	17 u
XhoI	10 u	70 u
SacI	5 u	35 u
XbaI	10 u	70 u

N.B. Use 3× excess for 1 h digests. For double digests choose a buffer compatible with both enzymes

Table 3.4. Sizes of vector ± inserts for digestions (kbp).

XhoI/XbaI cut	
Vector	1.0 + 3.0
Vector + Fd	1.7 + 3.0
Vector + Fab	2.4 + 3.0
Not I cut	
Vector	1.1 + 2.9
Vector + Fd	1.8 + 2.9
Vector + Fab	2.5 + 2.9
NheI/SpeI	
Vector + Fab	0.7 + 4.7

Protocol Part H – Vector preparation and insertion of PCR fragments

1. Inoculate a single colony of XL-1Blue infected with the vector (or vector + insert) from a plate or 10 ul from a frozen stock into a 10 ml culture of SB with 50 μg ml^{-1} carbenicillin (SB/Carb) and incubate overnight at 37°C on a shaker at 200 rpm.

2. Inoculate this 10 ml culture into 1 litre of SB/Carb and incubate overnight at 37°C on a shaker at 200 rpm.

3. Centrifuge at 4000 **g** for 10 min at 4°C.

4. Tip off the supernatant, add buffer P1 (Qiagen) as for 2 × Maxipreps and resuspend using the same pipette, then transfer to the column (Qiagen).

5. Follow the Qiagen protocol and at the completion wash both products each in 15 ml 70% EtOH (Centrifuge 4000 rpm in GS-6R or equivalent for 30 min to prevent loss of pellet).

6. Dry the tubes inverted for 5 min at room temperature.

7. Resuspend each product in 1mL DEPC (or nuclease free) water, aliquot (e.g. 25 μl per tube) and store at –20°C.

8. Digest 2 μl of the vector (or ~ 1–2 μg) preparation with 1 μl Not I (10 u μl^{-1}) in 42 μl DEPC treated water plus 5 μl Buffer H (10 ×) at 37°C for 1 h.

9. Load onto a 0.6% agarose gel and run for 1 h at 90 V (two bands should be evident at ~ 3000 and 1200 bp for vector without inserts).

10. Check the concentration of vector.

11. For restriction enzyme cleavage of vector to ligate Fd, digest 30 μg of vector with 90 u of SpeI and 270 u of XhoI, with 20 μl 10 × buffer (buffer 2, New England Biolabs; buffer H, Boehringer-Mannheim), in a total volume of 200 μl (made up with nuclease free water), for 3 h at 37°C.

12. Precipitate o/n at –20°C by adding 1/10 volume of 3 M NaAcetate (pH 5.2), 2.5 volumes of EtOH and 1 μl of glycogen.

13. Centrifuge at 15 000 rpm for 15 min in a microcentrifuge and wash in 1 ml of cold 70% EtOH.

14. Dissolve in 100 μl sterile nuclease free water and gel purify in 0.6% agarose.

15. Excise the 4700 bp band and recover the DNA by electroelution or silica glass beads.

16. Check the concentration of the cut vector.

17. Ligate cut Fd at a molar ratio of 1:2 (vector to insert) or 2 μg of cut vector to 0.7 μg of cut Fd in a total volume of 100 μl with 800 u of T4 ligase (New England BioLabs (NEB) # 202S) in ligase buffer (NEB)) at 16°C, overnight. Precipitate the ligation mix at –20°C, for at least 1 h, after adding ethanol to 70% (vol./vol.), then centrifuge at 14 000 **g**, in a microcentrifuge, for 15 min. When the DNA is completely dry, dissolve in 200 μl of nuclease free water.

18. Electroporate (pulse at 2.5 kV, i.e. 12.5 kV in a 0.2 cm gap cuvette for ~4.2 s) an equal amount of religated vector (~2.7 μg) and unligated (control for background) vector each into 300 μl of electrocompetent (>10^9 per g pUC19) *E. coli* XL1-Blue.

19. Flush the electroporation cuvette, first with 1 ml and then with 2 ml of SOC and incubate immediately in this 3 ml of SOC for 1 h at 37°C in a shaker (200 rpm).

20. Add 10 ml of prewarmed (37°C) SB (20 μg/ml carbenicillin (Carb) and 10 μg ml^{-1} tetracycline (Tet)) and immediately titrate transformants by plating 20 μl, 1 μl and 0.1 μl on LB plates (100 μg ml^{-1} Carb).

21. Incubate for 1 h at 37°C on a shaker.

22. Add this culture to 100 ml SB (50 μg ml^{-1} Carb, 10 μg ml^{-1} Tet) and incubate overnight at 37°C, on a shaker.

23. Prepare the phagemid DNA with Fd insert as for steps 3–10 above.

24. For insertion of digested light chain, repeat steps 11–23 above using 150 u SacI and 270 u XbaI (buffer 4, New England Biolabs; buffer A, Boehringer-Mannheim) in place of XhoI and SpeI.

Protocol Part I – Packaging of phagemid library for panning

1. After ligation of the second insert (usually light chain) and transformation of the library (electroporation) into XL1-Blue, the phagemid DNA must be packaged for expression of Fab on the head of the phage particles.

2. Electroporate the 20 μl of ligation mix, diluted 1/5 in DEPC water to 100 μl, as in Part H. step 18 above.

3. Flush the electroporation cuvette, first with 1 ml and then with 2 ml of SOC and incubate immediately in this 3 ml of SOC for 1 h at 37°C in a shaker (200 rpm).

4. Add 10 ml of prewarmed (37°C) SB (20 μg ml^{-1} carbenicillin (Carb) and 10 μg ml^{-1} tetracycline (Tet)) and immediately titrate transformants by plating 20 μl, 1 μl, and 0.1 μl on LB plates (100 μg ml^{-1} carbenicillin (Carb)).

5. Incubate the 10 ml culture for 1 h at 37°C on a shaker.

6. Add this 10 ml culture to 100 ml SB (50 μg ml^{-1} Carb, 10 μg ml^{-1} Tet) and incubate for 1 h at 37°C on a shaker.
7. Add helper phage VCSM13 (total of 10^{12} pfu).
8. Incubate on the shaker for 2 h at 37°C.
9. Add kanamycin to 70 mg ml^{-1} and incubate on a shaker overnight at 30°C.
10. Spin cells down at 6000 **g** (e.g. 6000 rpm in Sorvall GS3 or Beckman JA-10), at 4°C for 15 min and add to the supernatant 1.6 g PEG 8000, 1.2 g NaCl per 40 ml, mix and dissolve (or alternatively add 5 ml of 20% PEG/2.5 M NaCl per 20 ml of culture supernatant).
11. Precipitate phage on ice for 30 min.
12. Spin down precipitate at about 14 000 **g** (e.g. 11 000 rpm (Sorvall SS34 or Beckman JA-20) or 9 000 rpm (Sorvall GS3 or Beckman JA-10)), for 20 min at 4°C and discard the supernatant.
13. Resuspend pellet in 2ml PBS/1 % BSA, centrifuge for 5 min 14 000 rpm in a microcentrifuge and store the supernatant at 4°C (for long-term storage add NaN_3).
14. Titer this expanded phage suspension by infecting 50 μl volumes of XL1-Blue cells (OD_{600} = 0.5) with 1 μl of 10^{-3}, 10^{-6} and 10^{-8} dilutions of phage suspension, for 15 min at room temperature and plating on LB/Carb plates (incubate overnight at 37°C).

Note

For panning packaged phagemid must be prepared freshly on the day of panning, due to proteolytic cleavage of the Fab from the head of the phage on storage.

Protocol Part J – Repackaging of phagemid library

1. Infect 10 ml of freshly cultured XL1-Blue (OD_{600} = 0.5) with the packaged phagemid (~10^{11} total cfu) and incubate for 15 min at 37°C.
2. Add this to 100 ml SB (50 μg ml^{-1} Carb, 10 μg ml^{-1} Tet) and incubate for 1 h at 37°C on a shaker.
3. Add helper phage VCSM13 (total of 10^{12} pfu).
4. Incubate on the shaker for 2 h at 37°C.
5. Add kanamycin to 70 mg ml^{-1} and incubate on a shaker overnight at 30°C.
6. Harvest and titrate packaged phagemid as from step 10. above (Part G).

Protocol Part K – Panning for selection of clones producing antibody to specific antigens

1. Coat 4 ELISA plate wells overnight at 4°C with 50 or 25 μl of antigen (1 μg well^{-1}) solution in coating buffer (0.1 M bicarbonate pH 8.6).
2. Wash 6 × with H_2O.
3. Block by filling the wells completely with PBS/BSA (3%) and incubate in a humidified container for 1 h at 37°C then remove the liquid.

4. Add 50 μl phage suspension to each well (total of about 10^{11} pfu).
5. Incubate for 2 h at 37°C in humidified container.
6. Remove the phage, wash 10 × with PBS/Tween20 0.05%, incubating at room temperature for 5 min between washes.
7. Elute the phage by washing each of the 4 wells with 50 μl of elution buffer (0.1 M HCl (adjusted with glycine to pH 2.2)/BSA (1 mg ml^{-1}) and adding the eluent to 3 μl of 2 M Tris per 50 μl of elution buffer used. Pipette elution buffer up and down and scratch the well surface with the tip during this process.
8. Infect 2 ml of fresh XL-1 blue (OD_{600} = 0.5) with the eluted phage and incubate for 15 min at 37°C.
9. Add 10 ml of 37°C prewarmed SB (20 mg ml^{-1} Carb and 10 mg ml^{-1} Tet) and immediately titrate the eluted phage by plating (1 μl and 0.1 μl (10^{-4} and 10^{-5} dilution of total) on LB/Carb plates. Incubate the 10 ml culture for 1 h at 37°C on a shaker.
10. Add this 10 ml culture to 100 ml SB (50 μg ml^{-1} Carb and 10 μg ml^{-1} Tet) and incubate for 1 h at 37°C on a shaker.
11. Add helper phage VCSM13 (total of 10^{12} pfu).
12. Incubate on the shaker for 2 h at 37°C.
13. Add kanamycin to 70 mg ml^{-1} and incubate on a shaker o/n at 30°C.
14. Spin cells down at 6000 **g** at 4°C for 15 min and add to the supernatant 1.6 g PEG 8000, 1.2 g NaCl per 40 ml, mix and dissolve (or alternatively add 5 ml of 20% PEG/2.5 M NaCl per 20 ml of culture supernatant).
15. Precipitate phage on ice for 30 min.
16. Spin down precipitate at about 14 000 **g** for 20 min at 4°C and discard the supernatant.
17. Resuspend pellet in 2 ml PBS/1% BSA, centrifuge for 5 min at 14 000 **g** in a microcentrifuge and store the supernatant at 4°C (for long-term storage add NaN_3).
18. For subsequent panning reapply 50 μl of the above phagemid preparation to antigen coated wells (step 1) and add expanded phage from the previous panning.
19. After the fourth panning count the colonies and if less than a 100-fold increase eluted phage/applied phage (or relative yield) has been obtained over all 4 pannings, a fifth pan may be required (see *Table 3.1* for typical results).
20. From the expanded cultures of the last panning, make DNA from the *E. coli* cell pellet, using the Qiagen midi plasmid kit, for excision of the gene III DNA and religation to express soluble Fab.

Notes

Titer phage suspension by infecting 50 μl volumes of XL-1 blue cells (OD_{600} = 0.5) with 1 μl of 10^{-3}, 10^{-6} and 10^{-8} dilutions of phage suspension for 15 min at room temperature and plating on LB/Carb plates (incubate o/n at 37°C).

Remove 1–2 μl of the phagemid preparation after each panning and store in 20% glycerol at –80°C.

Protocol Part L – Production of soluble Fab after enrichment by panning

1. Collect the cell pellet from the last panning and prepare double stranded DNA (e.g. using the Qiagen midi plasmid kit).
2. Digest 10 μg of DNA with 30 u of SpeI and 100 u of NheI, with 20 μl 10 × buffer (buffer 2, New England Biolabs; buffer H, Boehringer-Mannheim), in a total volume of 200 μl (made up with nuclease free water), for 3 h at 37°C.
3. Add 40 μl of 6 × load buffer and run on a 0.6% agarose gel with 1 kb DNA marker.
4. Isolate the 4.7 kb band and purify by electroelution or silica beads (e.g. Qiaex).
5. Quantitate the DNA (EtBr plate or OD260) and religate 2 μg of DNA with T4 ligase (2 μg of vector with gene III DNA excised in a total volume of 100 μl with 800 u of T4 ligase (New England BioLabs (NEB) # 202S) in ligase buffer (NEB)) at 16°C, overnight. Precipitate the ligation mix at –20°C, for at least 1 h, after adding ethanol to 70% (vol/vol), then centrifuge at 14 000 **g** in a microcentrifuge, for 15 min. When the DNA is completely dry, dissolve in 200 μl of nuclease free water.
6. Transform 100 μl of this ligation mix into 300 μl of freshly thawed electrocompetent XL1-Blue cells as described for steps 18–21, *Protocol Part H*. NB. Transform an equal amount of cut vector to check for background in the transformation.
7. Plate 100 μl of the transformation mix in SB onto LB/Carb plates (100 μg ml^{-1} Carb) and incubate overnight at 37°C.
8. If the background (i.e. number of colonies) for the cut vector is at least 10-fold lower, pick colonies into 10 ml of SB/20 mM $MgCl_2$/50 μg ml^{-1} Carb and incubate at 37°C for ~ 6 h (OD_{600} ~ 1.5), then induce by addition of IPTG to a final concentration of 1 mM. After induction with IPTG, cultures should be incubated at 30°C overnight.
9. At the time of inoculation of Fab cultures, the same colonies should also be streaked out onto LB/Carb plates and these incubated at 37°C overnight.
10. Centrifuge cultures at 1500 **g** and tip off supernatants (the pellet generally contains a greater amount of Fab).
11. Resuspend the cell pellet in 0.2 ml PBS/0.2 mM PMSF/0.01% NaN_3 and freeze thaw the cells three times.
12. Pellet the cell debris by centrifugation at 14 000 **g**, for 10 min, in a microcentrifuge, transfer the supernatants to fresh tubes and test them by ELISA, for binding of Fab to the antigen(s) used for panning.

Notes

ELISA detection of soluble Fab-producing clones

The ELISA assay is not described here, but is analogous to the ELISA assay for detection of monoclonal antibody, described in *Chapter 2*. The detection reagent is antibody/enzyme conjugate (antihuman $F(ab')_2$-alkaline phosphatase) (e.g. Pierce Cat. No. 31312 at 1/500 in PBS) and the substrate is Sigma phosphatase substrate Cat. No. 104–105 in 5 ml alkaline phosphatase staining buffer.

Fab clones showing a high differential OD in ELISA for the positive antigen, compared to the control negative (e.g. 5 × – 10 ×), should be streaked on LB/Carb plates to isolate single colonies again at this stage. This obviates the loss of a positive clone from a mixed colony, by overgrowth with a negative or polyreactive Fab clone.

These same clones exhibiting a high differential for positive versus negative antigen, should be purified for titration with positive and negative antigens again, since crude periplasmic extracts are often cross-reactive.

Once purified Fab has been titrated and confirmed to have a similar pattern of reactivity as the original 10 ml culture product, a single colony from a freshly streaked overnight culture should be used for DNA isolation (e.g. Qiagen preparation) and for freezing as a glycerol stock (10% glycerol/LB broth).

The expected protein yield of Fab varies from 10 μg to 4 mg l^{-1}.

Protocol 3.2

Purification of human Fab

Procedure

1. Use freshly streaked plates to set up a 10 ml overnight culture (SB/20 mM $MgCl_2$/50 μg Carb/ml (SB/Mg/Carb)) for each liter to be inoculated, or if taking inoculum from a freshly streaked single colony use a full loop of inoculum for 1 liter of culture
2. Use the whole 10 ml overnight culture to inoculate the 1 liter of SB/Mg/Carb (10 ml 2 M $MgCl_2$ and 0.5 ml of Carb (100 mg ml^{-1})).
3. Set up 1 l culture early in the day and induce with 1 mM IPTG at the end of the day (or OD600 = 0.6), then incubate at 30°C on a shaker (200 rpm), overnight.
4. Harvest the cells the next morning.
5. Centrifuge at 4000 ***g*** for 30 min at 4°C, decant the supernatant and keep the cell pellet.
6. Sonicate the pellet for 2 min at 50% after resuspending the pellet from each liter culture in 25 ml PBS/0.01% azide/0.2 mM PMSF. Alternatively freeze/thaw the pellet × 3 in PBS/azide/PMSF.
7. Centrifuge the sonicated or freeze/thawed pellet (~30 ml) at 11 000–13 000 ***g*** for 40 min at 4°C.
8. Filter the supernatant from the sonicated or freeze/thawed pellet using first 0.45 μm then 0.22 μm filters.
9. Store the supernatant from the sonicated pellet (with sodium azide (0.01%) or Thimerosal (0.005%)), at 4°C to prevent precipitation on thawing.
10. Purify on Protein G or anti-Fab column (see *Protocol 2.7, Chapter 2*).
11. After neutralizing with 1/10 vol. 1 M Tris pH 9 and pooling the fractions containing the Fab peak, concentrate to about 1 ml per 25–30 ml pellet using a Centriprep 30 (Amicon Cat. # 4306), and check by SDS-PAGE for a single band at ~50 000 Da (nonreduced). Filter through a 0.2 μm sterile filter and store at 4°C.
12. If fractions have more than one band (e.g. due to dissociation of the light chain and heavy chain fragment) then run them on a 2 ml Mono S column, pool fractions with a single band (50 000 Da), concentrate as above and wash with buffer of choice (e.g. Dulbecco's PBS).
13. Filter (0.2 μm) and store at 4°C.

The Basics

Chapter 4

Applications of monoclonal antibodies to the study of molecules in solution

D A Brooks

1. Introduction

This chapter describes the use of monoclonal antibodies to study lysosomal proteins and their associated disease states, to illustrate the range of applications of monoclonal antibodies in the study of soluble molecules. A brief overview of the cellular organelles involved in protein processing and trafficking pathways for lysosomal proteins is presented first, to set the scene.

1.1 The vacuolar network

During synthesis, protein destined for the intracellular vacuole system and the secretory pathway are translocated into the lumen of the endoplasmic reticulum. These include integral membrane and lumenal proteins of the endoplasmic reticulum, the Golgi apparatus, the endosomal network, lysosomes and those proteins trafficking via the trans-Golgi network destined for extracellular secretion and the cell surface (*Figure 4.1*). Within the lumen of the endoplasmic reticulum proteins are folded and modified in a concerted process catalyzed by molecular chaperones. The primary role of the endoplasmic reticulum is to prevent incorrect association of peptide sequences or motifs and to promote the assembly of polypeptides and formation of correct secondary, tertiary and quaternary structure. N-linked glycosylation also occurs in the endoplasmic reticulum.

The Golgi complex (*Figure 4.1*) is a specialized compartment for glycoprotein processing and for synthesizing and attaching oligosaccharides to protein, and controls protein traffic and sorting to either vesicular compartments (e.g. endosome-lysosome proteins), or the cell surface (e.g. cell surface and secretory proteins).

1.2 Analysis of vacuolar network proteins using immunochemistry

Antibodies are frequently used as specific probes to facilitate protein identification in complex mixtures. Some examples of the use of immunochemistry for protein analysis (and in particular the use of

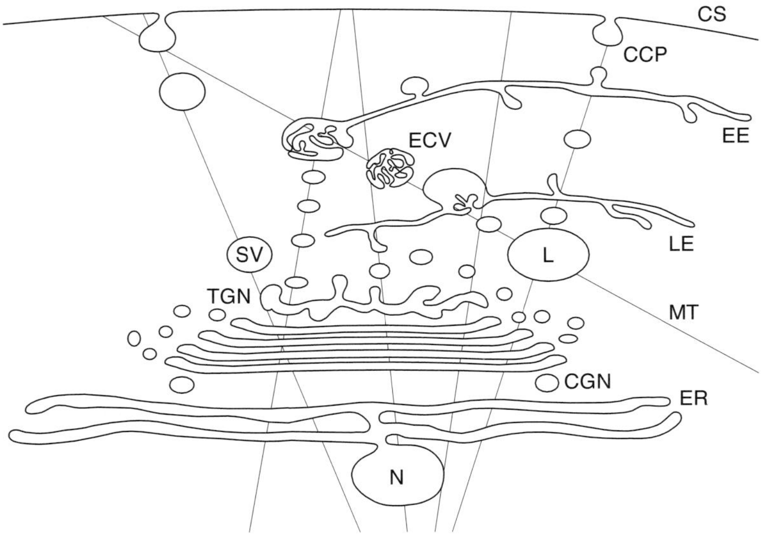

Figure 4.1

Elements of the vacuolar network. Proteins destined for the vacuolar network and cell surface (CS) are synthesized in the endoplasmic reticulum (ER) then traffic to the Golgi apparatus for further processing (CGN: cis Golgi network). At the trans-Golgi network (TGN) proteins are sorted for traffic to either the secretory pathway (SV, secretory vesicles: default pathway) or the endosome-lysosome system (EE, early endosome; ECV, endosome carrier vesicle; LE, late endosome; L, lysosome). Internalization of molecules from the cell surface and extracellular milieu into the vacuolar network via clathrin coated pits (CCP) and vesicular transport. Vesicles of the vacuolar network are arranged on and trafficked via microtubules (MT) which extend throughout the cellular cytoplasm.

monoclonal antibodies) follow. Quantitative immunoassays are usually developed to measure the concentration of a specific protein of interest, and often form the basis of diagnostic tests used in the analysis of patient samples. The purification of a molecule by immunoaffinity chromatography allows more detailed study, for example amino acid sequence analysis, and application of the molecule, including treatment of patients. The specific antigen binding capacity of antibodies can also be used to capture and analyse the protein of interest, facilitating, for example, detailed enzyme kinetic analysis by removing the protein from contaminants. Antibodies may also be used to dissect the molecular forms or polypeptide subunit structure of a protein and to probe the conformation of a protein. Antibodies can be used to specifically immunoprecipitate a protein and this has been used to study the intracellular biogenesis of proteins. When used in conjunction with radiolabelling, immunoprecipitation can be used to study protein synthesis, and subsequent glyco-processing or proteolytic processing events. For vacuolar network proteins this strategy has been used extensively to follow the maturation of proteins, allowing dissection of the many intracellular protein modification steps required for their function.

In this chapter the use of some core immunochemistry techniques is described with reference to the study of vacuolar network proteins. Protocols are included for selected techniques.

2. ELISA (enzyme linked immuno-adsorbent assay)

Homogenous immunoassays refer to the attachment of antigen to a solid phase (e.g. ELISA plate), followed by immune detection (in this chapter reference is made mainly to the detection of proteins but this methodology could equally apply to other antigens). This detection may either be by direct ELISA (*Figure 4.2*), where the antibody is labeled with an enzyme or fluorophore, or by indirect ELISA (*Figure 4.2*) which uses first a specific primary antibody then a secondary anti-antibody which is labelled and acts as the detection step. Heterogenous immunoassays (also referred to as sandwich or capture ELISAs) use two separate antibody reagents to the antigen, the first of which is attached to the solid phase to capture the antigen, while the second antibody is used for the detection step. Again the detection step may be either direct or indirect. ELISA may be used for the

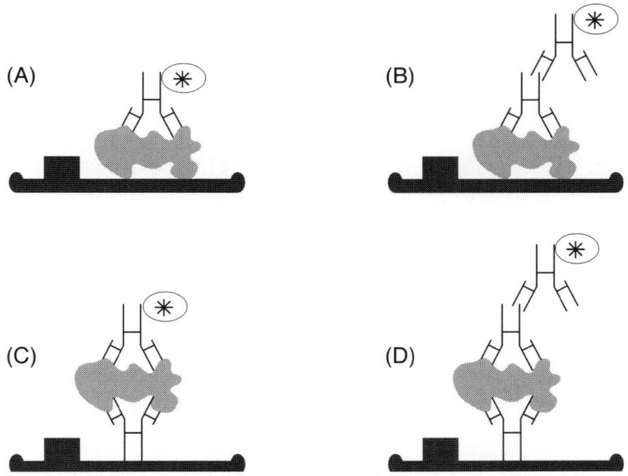

Figure 4.2

Immunoassays: homogenous, heterogenous, direct and indirect ELISA. At the base of each of the figures A–D is a representation of a solid phase (e.g. ELISA plate well). The solid black square indicates the use of a blocking solution of protein to coat nonspecific reactive sites on the ELISA plate (solid phase), following attachment of either the antigen (A and B; homogenous ELISA) or the antibody molecules (C and D; capture antibody in the heterogenous ELISA). (A) Homogenous immunoassay using a direct detection method (label attached to the primary antibody). (B) Homogenous immunoassay using an indirect detection method (label attached to the second antibody). (C) Heterogenous immunoassay using a direct detection method (one antibody for the capture step and another labelled antibody for the detection step). (D) Heterogenous immunoassay using an indirect detection method [one antibody for the capture step, another antibody for the primary detection and a labelled anti-antibody which is used to visualize the reaction (N.B. this labelled anti-antibody must not react with the capture antibody)]. In both A and B the protein of interest competes with other proteins in solution, for binding to the solid phase. In C and D the protein of interest is selectively purified away from contaminant proteins.

detection and analysis of an antigen, or conversely for the analysis of antibody responses to antigen

2.1 Advantages and disadvantages of homogenous and heterogenous ELISA

Relatively pure antigen is required for homogenous ELISA to be effective. For complex mixtures, the antigen of interest must compete with other molecules for the finite number of binding sites, during attachment to the solid phase. Improved detection is therefore achieved with increasing purity of the antigen. Homogenous ELISAs are best applied to qualitative detection of an antigen. For example, during purification procedures the analysis of a specific protein by ELISA obviates the need for activity analysis to trace the protein of interest. Similarly, homogenous ELISA can be applied for further analysis of a purified protein (e.g. to study interactions with another protein or in immunoblot analysis, as described in the section on immunoblotting).

Capture ELISAs overcome the problems of abundance and purity by using a capture step to first purify the molecule of interest away from contaminants. These assays are therefore suitable for antigen quantification, as they can detect a single protein in, for example, a cellular protein extract. Heterogenous ELISAs are suited to routine analysis of a specific protein, especially where a cellular protein is being studied and purification is not being undertaken. Importantly, they also allow the detection and analysis of proteins which do not have a catalytic activity. Heterogenous assays are particularly useful for the quantitative analysis of a specific protein in a complex protein mixture. A Protocol for ELISA for the detection of antibody is given in *Chapter 2*; this protocol can readily be adapted for detection and quantitative analysis of antigen.

Capture ELISA requires reagents which detect at least two spatially separated epitopes on the antigen. Typically the capture step may be achieved with a polyclonal antibody raised in one species (e.g. goat or rabbit) and the detection step can utilize either a polyclonal antibody from another species or preferably a monoclonal antibody. The use of two monoclonal antibodies in capture ELISAs gives the best specificity, but is associated with some problems. The capture of proteins using monoclonal antibodies is far less efficient than capture with polyclonal antibodies. Monoclonal antibodies generally react with a single site (epitope) on the target protein, compared to the multiple site reactivity of polyclonal antibodies. Capture efficiency is also dependent on the affinity of the monoclonal antibody. Polyclonal antibodies are mixtures which are likely to contain antibodies of high affinity, whilst a particular monoclonal antibody may or may not have adequate affinity. In indirect ELISA, the monoclonal antibodies used for capture and detection must not be from the same species, as the detection antibody will recognize the capture antibody. This problem can be overcome by using a direct ELISA detection step, but necessitates labeling of the monoclonal antibody used for the detection step.

The sensitivity of ELISA detection is highly dependent on the enzyme or fluorophore. Commonly used enzymes for ELISA detection include β-galactosidase, alkaline phosphatase and horseradish peroxidase. The sensitivity of antibody probes using these markers can be improved by signal amplification and frequently utilize complexes of biotinylated antibody and streptavidin linked to enzyme to increase the amount of enzyme recruited to each antigen site.

In ELISAs, a standard curve produced using an enzyme reagent is normally sigmoid, reflecting limited enzyme detection at very low levels, a linear range of optimal detection and a plateau of reactivity which reflects saturation enzyme kinetics. Time-resolved fluorimetry using lanthanide chelates offers an improved linear range for detection and an increased sensitivity compared to enzyme detection (Diamandis, 1988). Lanthanides tend to have limited background problems due to the large Stokes shift between excitation and emission wavelengths (340 nm to 614 nm for Europium). This allows efficient separation of the specific signal from scatter and interfering background fluorescence (usually at 400–600 nm). In time-resolved fluorescence, the increased duration of the lanthanide signal (10–1000 ms) compared to the time for the decay of background fluorescence (1–20 ms), also allows the detection event to be removed in time from the excitation event. Together, these factors provide a very high signal to noise ratio. An additional advantage of time resolved fluorescence detection is the ability to analyze multiple lanthanide elements (due to their different fluorescence properties), in the same assay (e.g. attached to different antibodies reacting with different analytes), allowing dual antibody detection in the same assay. The lanthanide chelate is usually dissociated for the detection procedure, giving enhanced signal. This assay procedure is called DELFIA (dissociation-enhanced lanthanide fluoroimmunoassay) and is used routinely in screening programs, such as newborn screening for inherited disorders of metabolism, because of its high sensitivity and reliability.

2.2 Illustration of application of ELISA in quantitative analysis of enzymes

Enzymes may be analyzed through the determination of enzymic activity and kinetics. However, for proteins which do not have catalytic activity, or for which assays have not been developed, antibody provides an alternative analytical method. In addition, the characterization of immunoreactive protein is ideal when analyzing proteins which are functionally defective. Thus, the question of whether a genetic deficiency state is due to lack of protein production or to synthesis of a functionally defective protein can be resolved. Moreover, multiple protein epitopes can be analysed by using different monoclonal antibodies, giving a picture of the structural aberration for the defective protein. Antibodies for this purpose may be against linear sequence epitopes (see section on epitope mapping) or against conformational epitopes, which reflect the protein's primary structure or secondary-tertiary-quaternary structure, respectively.

Lysosomal storage disorder patients have been characterized immunochemically, showing that most patients have low levels of mutant protein. Two lysosomal storage disorders, mucopolysaccharidosis type I (MPS I) and mucopolysaccharidosis type VI (MPS VI) have been analyzed by immunoquantification of cell extracts and demonstrate only low levels of immunoreactive protein, with less than 5% of that observed in normal controls. In MPS VI patients the 4-sulfatase protein detected is structurally altered, as determined by the number of missing or modified protein epitopes, and the degree of modification shows some correlation to the severity of clinical presentation. This was demonstrated using conformation sensitive monoclonal antibodies in an immunoquantification assay. The most severe MPS VI patients either have no immunodetectable protein or very low levels of protein with few detected epitopes, suggesting greater structural aberration. Radiolabel-immunoprecipitation studies show normal synthesis of mutant protein for most patients (see section on immunoprecipitation and radiolabel synthesis/processing). These findings lead to the hypothesis that mutant protein does not fold correctly and is recognized and degraded in the endoplasmic reticulum, shortly after synthesis, by a quality control process.

For both MPS I and MPS VI patient samples, some protein epitopes correlate with clinical severity. This type of correlation may be expected, as the level of structural alteration in a protein will influence enzyme function and thus disease severity. However, these markers are not absolute indicators of disease severity; some severely affected patients may have detectable protein (e.g. where enzyme is not properly localized or targeted to the lysosome), while some mildly affected patients may have no immunodetectable protein (e.g. due to missing or modified epitopes). This again reflects the need for a panel of diagnostic markers for effective protein detection and thus clinical phenotype prediction.

An exception to the trend described above involved an MPS I patient who was identified with at least six times the normal level of α-L-iduronidase protein (Brooks *et al.*, 1992) suggesting a mutation which resulted in a stable but catalytically inactive protein. This alteration in the α-L-iduronidase molecule must be structurally minor as the protein is neither recognized and retained for degradation by the endoplasmic reticulum, nor unstable in the lysosome. These studies highlight the need to use an array of immunochemical and cell biological tools to dissect complex systems.

3. Protein epitope delineation

The exquisite specificity of monoclonal antibodies results from their ability to bind to a precise antigenic determinant on a protein. Epitope mapping and epitope delineation are terms used for the process of identifying the specific epitope recognized by an antibody. The procedure described in this section allows the identification of linear sequence peptide epitopes and the location of these epitopes in relation to structural elements, including protein subunits, the enzyme active site and carbohydrate attachment sites.

ELISA of native protein (fully folded with conformational epitopes) versus denatured protein (linearized to expose linear sequence epitopes) is recommended prior to epitope mapping. Reactivity to denatured protein generally signals the recognition of either a linear sequence epitope or a carbohydrate epitope. Linear protein epitopes can be mapped by determining their reactivity with synthetic peptides (as described in this section), while carbohydrate epitopes may be mapped by similar studies using carbohydrates.

Strategies for epitope mapping of antibodies have been commercialized (e.g. Chiron Mimotopes) and use ELISA. Short peptide sequences, from the protein of interest, are synthesized onto polyethylene or polypropylene pins. The complete linear sequence of the protein is synthesized as 10–15mer peptides, with overlaps of 5–8 amino acids, to avoid epitope splitting and to represent all possible polypeptide epitopes. The antibody to be tested is then reacted by ELISA with the peptides on the pins (i.e. the pins become the solid phase and can be inserted into ELISA plate wells for incubations with the antibody detection reagents).

Once the antibody reactive linear sequences have been identified, the epitopes can be mapped onto the linear sequence of the protein. Furthermore, if the crystal structure of the protein has been determined, the antibody epitopes identified can be mapped onto molecular drawings of the molecule, revealing surface or internal molecular location of the epitope. This may be particularly useful in ascertaining the immunogenicity of a molecule and the specific location of high and low immunogenicity regions of the protein. For lysosomal proteins studied in the author's laboratory, this has been particularly important for studying immune reactivity to replacement proteins used to treat patients with genetic diseases.

Enzyme replacement therapy has been identified as an effective treatment strategy for patients with genetic disease such as lysosomal storage disorder. However, repeated infusions can result in an immune response to the replacement protein. Antibody reactivity to linear sequence epitopes on the replacement proteins have been mapped to define background immune reactivity to the proteins and the immune response to the infused proteins.

Monoclonal antibodies to these enzymes have also been epitope mapped. A monoclonal antibody to the lysosomal enzyme α-L-iduronidase, which has proven to be ideal for both immunoblotting and immunopurification, was studied (*Figure 4.3*). The epitope appeared to be located on surface residues of the α-L-iduronidase protein between two N-linked glycosylation sites (used in lysosomal targeting, *Figure 4.4*). This indicated that the epitope was accessible and confirmed its linear sequence reactivity.

4. Assays of antibody-bound antigen

Proteins with an enzyme activity can be bound to an antibody, then assayed for their specific activity. This type of assay has been referred to as an enzyme immunobinding assay (*Figure 4.5*). Immunobinding assays are a useful adjunct to ELISA analysis of purified protein, and also aid in assessing the specific reactivity of an antibody with an enzyme. In this system the antibody purifies the protein of interest away from contaminants in the capture-wash steps, providing an optimal system for enzyme activity assays and kinetic studies.

Either polyclonal or monoclonal antibodies can be attached to a solid phase for the capture step. For polyclonal antibodies this usually requires purified antibody (e.g. protein G purified antibody) or even better affinity

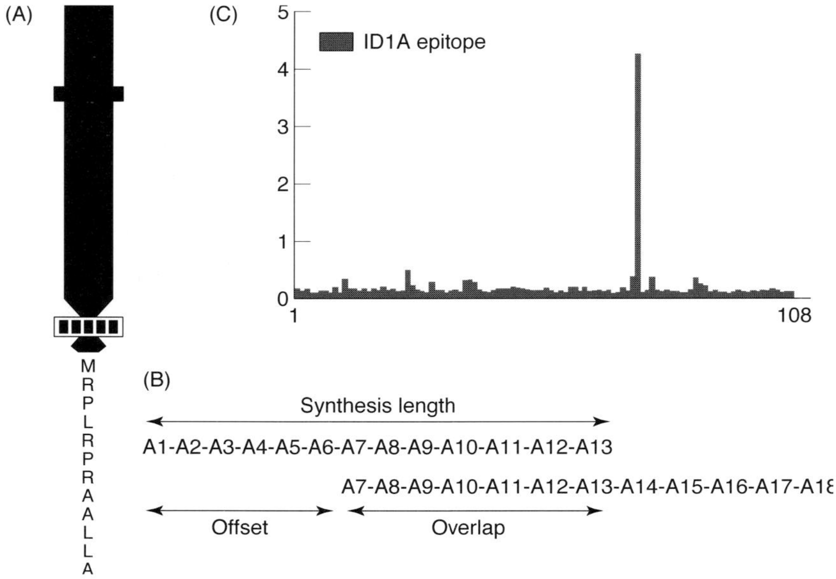

Figure 4.3

Strategy for epitope mapping of monoclonal antibodies using peptide pin plates. Epitope mapping of a monoclonal antibody to the lysosomal protein α-L-iduronidase was achieved using peptide pin plates. (A) Diagrammatic representation of a peptide pin, with the synthetic peptide attached to one end. (B) The strategy for the synthesis of overlapping α-L-iduronidase peptides, which is designed to avoid missing epitopes and to prevent epitope splitting. (C) The ELISA reactivity of the monoclonal antibody to synthetic peptides from the lysosomal protein α-L-iduronidase.

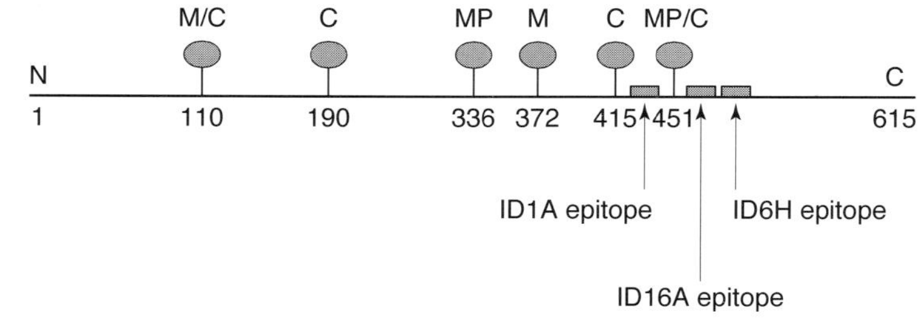

Figure 4.4

Monoclonal antibody epitope location on a lysosomal protein. Figure represents the linear protein sequence of the lysosomal protein α-L-iduronidase (615 amino acids). The position and nature of the N-linked oligosaccharides on α-L-iduronidase have been marked (M depicts high mannose oligosaccharide; C depicts complex oligosaccharide; MP depicts mannose-6-phosphorylated oligosaccharide) and the position of three separate monoclonal antibody linear sequence epitopes are shown (ID1A, ID6H and ID16A).

purified antibody (ie. antibody purified by chromatography on a specific antigen column, which results in a high concentration of the specific antibody being attached to the solid phase). Crude monoclonal antibody culture supernatants can be used in immunobinding assays, by using an

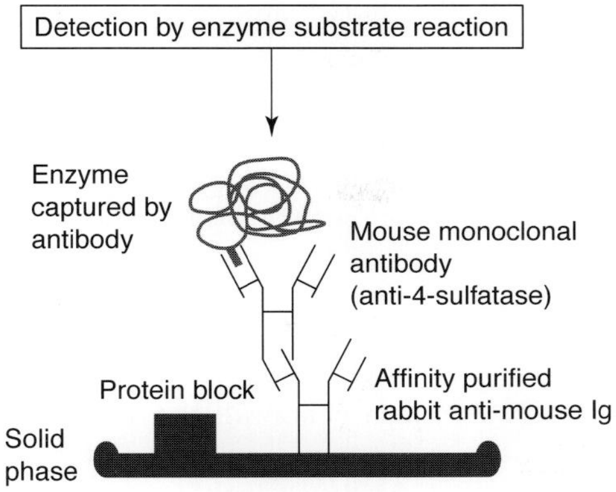

Figure 4.5

Immunobinding assay for capture and assay of enzyme activity. A capture antibody (affinity purified rabbit anti-mouse immunoglobulin) is shown attached to a solid phase (ELISA plate well). The solid black square indicates the use of a blocking solution of protein to coat non-specific reactive sites on the ELISA plate following attachment of the capture antibody. A mouse monoclonal antibody which reacts specifically with the lysosomal protein 4-sulfatase is bound to the capture antibody. The latter antibody is used to, in turn, capture the lysosomal enzyme, which can then be detected by an enzyme substrate reaction.

anti-antibody capture reagent to attach to the solid phase prior to adsorption of the monoclonal antibody. Monoclonal antibody usually detects a single determinant on the target molecule, whereas polyclonal antibodies tend to be better capture reagents due to their polyspecific nature. On the other hand, polyclonal antibodies may have reactivities which bind to and interfere with the activity of the enzyme being analyzed (i.e. active site antibodies). Monoclonal antibodies are site specific and can be tested for their effect on enzyme specific activity.

The bound enzyme is detected by assaying with a suitable substrate. A specific assay for the lysosomal enzyme N-acetylgalactosamine-4-sulfatase (4-sulfatase) has been developed and uses a monoclonal antibody to specifically bind and separate 4-sulfatase (arylsulfatase B) from other sulfatases. The bound enzyme is then incubated with methylumbelliferyl sulfate substrate for detection or enzyme kinetic studies. A similar strategy has been used to specifically assay human 4-sulfatase in tissue samples from cats in which enzyme distribution was studied following enzyme infusion experiments. This required the separation of human and cat 4-sulfatase and utilized a monoclonal antibody which detected human but not cat 4-sulfatase for the capture step. The unique specificity of monoclonal antibodies can therefore be used to separate either different forms of proteins or the same protein from different species, before enzyme activity analysis.

5. Immunoaffinity chromatography (see *Protocol 4.1*)

Polyclonal antisera have been used to purify proteins; however, in general, these reagents are not ideal for immunopurification due to the presence of varying affinities and cross-reacting antibodies. Antibodies of very high affinity or avidity can require excessively denaturing conditions for elution. Monoclonal antibodies have a single specificity and affinity/avidity, and antibodies with suitable properties can be selected and used for immunopurification, allowing the unique binding site of the antibody to act as a specific ligand for the protein of interest.

The essential features of an immunoaffinity chromatography matrix include a covalent linkage between the support matrix and the antibody to prevent leakage during chromatography, an antibody-matrix linkage which does not alter the specificity of the antibody upon coupling, a spacer arm which prevents steric inhibition of the antibody interaction by the matrix, an inert matrix to reduce nonspecific interactions and, finally, a matrix which is rigid under chromatography conditions.

Elution is often the most difficult step in immunoaffinity chromatography. To achieve high yield and purity an elution protocol must not denature the eluted antigen but must effectively disrupt the antigen antibody interaction. The elution conditions must be optimized for each antibody interaction. Low pH elution has proved to be effective for lysosomal enzymes (see Gibson *et al.*, 1987; Clements *et al.*, 1989; *Figure 4.6*).

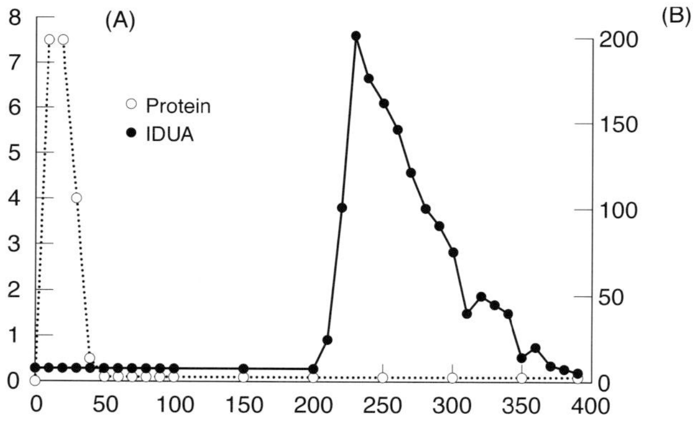

Figure 4.6

Immunopurification by monoclonal antibody affinity chromatography and immunoblot detection of the lysosomal protein α-L-iduronidase. (A) Human liver α-L-iduronidase was partially purified by blue-A agarose column chromatography (Clements et al., *1989), then purified to homogeneity by ID1A monoclonal antibody immunoaffinity chromatography. Protein (-○-○-, left axis, A_{280} × 10^{-1}) and α-L-iduronidase enzyme activity (-●-●-, right axis, nmol/min/ml × 10^{-6}). (B) Immunoblot detection of α-L-iduronidase using the monoclonal antibody ID1A. ID1A detects most of the high molecular weight polypeptide subunits associated with the mature α-L-iduronidase protein (see* Figure 4.8 *for proteolytic clipping events for α-L-iduronidase and the theoretical reactivity of ID1A with these polypeptide subunits). The molecular weights of the bands detected on the immunoblot are from top to bottom: 74, 65 (major), 60, 49, 44 kDa (N.B. the 78 kDa precursor is usually only a minor band in preparations of liver enzyme as it is rapidly processed and is therefore not detected by ID1A on the immunoblot).*

6. Western blotting (see *Protocol 4.2*)

Immunoblotting is suited primarily to the detection of denatured or linear sequence epitopes on proteins. Immunoblotting may be carried out on proteins simply blotted onto a substrate material such as nitrocellulose, or after electrophoretic separation of proteins and transfer to the substrate material. The former procedure is referred to as dot- or slot-blotting, the latter as western blotting. Dot- and slot-blotting are essentially variations of ELISA and are not discussed further here. Western blotting is a useful technique for identifying the protein target of an antibody. It is also a powerful technique for the subunit analysis of proteins or for the detection of proteolytic or other processing modifications, which result in multiple forms of a protein. This is well illustrated in the analysis of the polypeptide species associated with the lysosomal enzyme α-L-iduronidase, where proteolytic processing is a normal part of the maturation of the protein (see *Figures 4.6* and *4.7*).

The major limitation of the technique is that only denatured protein can be readily analyzed due to the conditions required for the first step of the electrophoretic separation. Antibodies which are suitable for western blotting are usually directed either towards primary protein structure (i.e. linear sequence) or to very stable secondary structures (e.g. β-turns or structures stabilized by covalent linkages) or in some cases to carbohydrate epitopes. The production of antibodies suitable for western blotting is therefore favored by immunization protocols with denatured protein antigens.

Western blotting analysis of samples derived from inborn error of metabolism patients has given some insight into the protein consequences

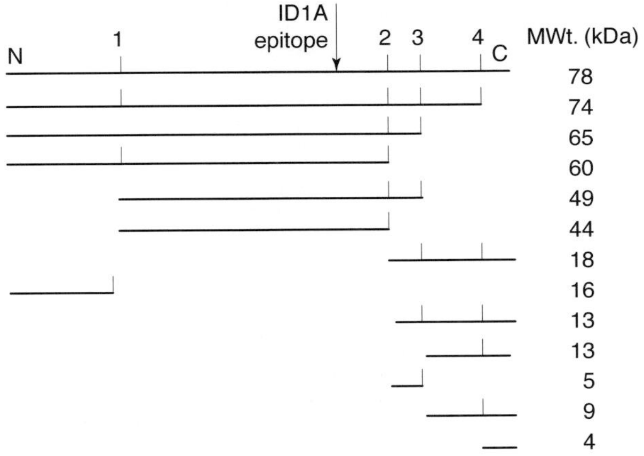

Figure 4.7

Polypeptide proteolytic processing of a lysosomal protein. The molecular size and proteolytic clip points of the α-L-iduronidase protein are shown relative to the ID1A monoclonal antibody epitope. The 78 kDa precursor molecule is synthesized in the ER, while the proteolytic clipping events are thought to occur in the endosome-lysosome system. N and C termini of the protein are shown. The potential proteolytic clip sites are numbered 1–4.

of gene mutations. Identification of processed forms of the same protein is particularly important when trying to discern a protein in a complex mixture and allows the identification of processed forms for further analysis (e.g. confirmation of peptide fragments or forms by sequence analysis).

7. Immunoprecipitation and radiolabel synthesis/processing (see *Protocol 4.3*)

Immunoprecipitation techniques can be used as an alternative to immunobinding assay and immunoaffinity chromatography and are applicable for most polyclonal antisera. For a monoclonal antibody which reacts with one epitope per protein molecule, immunoprecipitation requires the use of a second antibody to allow cross-linking or a solid phase to retrieve the antibody–antigen complex. Immunoprecipitation assays (using only antibody reagents) require titration of the antigen and antibody in order to form optimum precipitates and to avoid prozone phenomena (failure to precipitate due to antigen or antibody excess). A major drawback of precipitation reactions is the potential for nonspecific coprecipitation of proteins.

Immunoprecipitation is used frequently in conjunction with radiolabeling to study the synthesis and processing of proteins. Pulse radiolabel followed by short chase times in the absence of radiolabel can be used to identify specific points in the maturation of a protein as it traffics through the cellular processing machinery. Immunoprecipitation allows the recovery of the protein of interest from appropriate time windows, purifying it away from other labelled proteins. The labelled protein can then be analyzed by sodium dodecyl sulfate-polyacrylamide gel electrophoresis (SDS-PAGE) to define molecular sizes of polypeptide species, often reflecting the specific processing events. Detection is usually by autoradiography of the gel.

For example, synthesis of a glycosylated lysosomal polypeptide in the endoplasmic reticulum may be identified by [^{35}S]-cysteine [^{35}S]-methionine amino acid labeling of the protein (in the order of 10–20 min for most proteins). The labelled protein may then be traced as it traffics to the Golgi (further 20–30 min) where modification of its N-linked oligosaccharides may result in a size change. For lysosomal proteins, the N-linked oligosaccharides are mannose-6-phosphorylated in the Golgi, which signals routing to the lysosome. This can be detected by labeling with [^{32}P]-phosphate before recovery by immunoprecipitation. Traffic of lysosomal proteins through the endosome–lysosome network can often be detected by specific carbohydrate and protein processing events. Thus, lysosomal proteins are frequently proteolytically modified to form a mature lysosomal protein. Again after appropriate labeling and immunoprecipitation, these events can be characterized by molecular mass changes detected by SDS-PAGE and autoradiography.

The analysis of lysosomal proteins by immunoprecipitation/radiolabeling has demonstrated that in patients the mutant protein produced is handled in different ways by the cellular machinery. In some patients message instability results in reduced synthesis of protein. In many lysosomal storage disorder patients normal synthesis occurs but the endoplasmic reticulum quality control system recognizes the mutant protein as incorrectly folded and targets it for premature degradation. Some proteins are not modified correctly and are improperly targeted within the cell, reaching inappropriate destinations (resulting in either reduced activity, or activity at the wrong cellular location or in increased enzyme turnover). Each processing event can result in error. The complexity of many of these cell biological processes can be dissected using radiolabel–immunoprecipitation techniques. This can be further refined by the subcellular fractionation of specific cellular organelles (see the next section).

8. Immuno-organelle binding assays

Subcellular fractionation of cells is a powerful technique for the analysis of intracellular membrane bound, organellar proteins. The use of antibody to capture specific organelles provides a further level of sophistication for cell biology studies (*Figure 4.8*). Immune capture techniques potentially can provide very pure preparations of organelles, which are dependent only on the membrane associated proteins which comprise the outer surface of the organelle. The purified organelles can allow the study of internal enzyme components without organelle disruption, facilitating more appropriate enzyme kinetic studies, or the isolation and study of protein components which comprise the organelle.

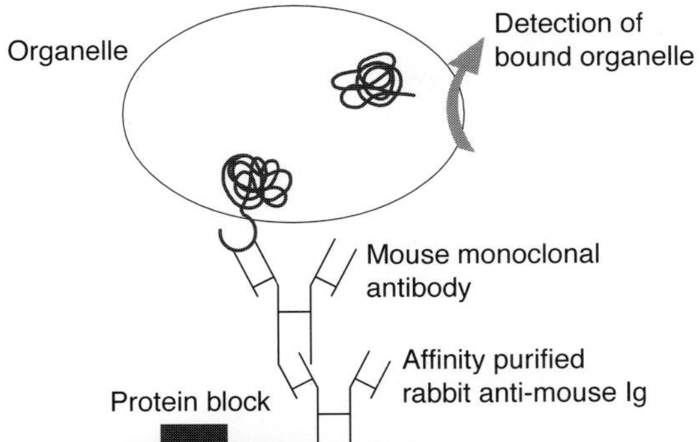

Figure 4.8

Organelle immunobinding assay. A capture antibody (affinity purified rabbit anti-mouse immunoglobulin) is shown attached to a solid phase (ELISA plate well). The solid black square indicates the use of a blocking solution of protein to coat non-specific reactive sites on the ELISA plate following attachment of the capture antibody. A mouse monoclonal antibody which reacts specifically with a membrane protein on the cytosolic side of the organelle to be bound (e.g. lysosomal membrane protein) is bound by the capture antibody. The monoclonal antibody is then used to capture organelles from subcellular fractions. The bound organelle can be detected by the reactivity of a specific enzyme, contained within the organelle of interest.

References

Brooks, D.A., McCourt, P.A.G., Gibson, G.J., Ashton, L.J., Shutter, M. and Hopwood, J.J. (1991) Analysis of N-acetylgalactosamine-4-sulfatase protein and kinetics in mucopolysaccharidosis type VI patients. *Am. J. Hum. Genet.* **48**, 710–719.

Brooks, D.A., Harper, G.S., Gibson, G.J., Ashton, L.J., McCourt, P.A.G., Taylor, J.A., Freeman, C., Clements, P.R., Hoffmann, J.W. and Hopwood, J.J. (1992) Hurler syndrome: a patient with abnormally high levels of α-L-iduronidase protein. *J. Biochem. Med. Metab. Biol.* **47**, 211–220.

Brooks, D.A., Bradford, T.M., Carlsson, S.R. and Hopwood, J.J. (1997) A membrane protein primarily associated with the lysosomal compartment. *Biochem. Biophys. Acta* **1327**, 162–170.

Clements, P.R., Brooks, D.A., McCourt, P.A.G. and Hopwood, J.J. (1989) Immunopurification and characterisation of human α-L-iduronidase with the use of monoclonal antibodies. *Biochem. J.* **259**, 199–208.

Diamandis, E.P. (1988) Immunoassays with time-resolved fluorescence spectroscopy: principles and applications. *Clin. Biochem.* **21**, 139–150.

Gibson, G., Saccone, G., Brooks, D., Clements, P. and Hopwood, J. (1987) Human N-acetylgalactosamine-4-sulphate sulphatase: purification, monoclonal antibody production, native and subunit M_r values. *Biochem. J.* **248**, 755–764.

Kornfeld, S. (1987) Trafficking of lysosomal enzymes. *FASEB J.* **1**, 462–468.

Laemmli, U.K. (1970) Cleavage of structural proteins during the assembly of the head of bacteriophage T4. *Nature,* **227**, 680–685.

Protocol 4.1

Immunoaffinity chromatography

Materials

Affi-Gel 10: Affi-Gel 10 from BioRad Laboratories (use according to the manufacturer's instructions)

Mouse monoclonal antibody: 4-S F58.3 high affinity monoclonal antibody specific for the human lysosomal enzyme *N*-acetylgalactosamine-4-sulfatase (4-sulfatase: Brooks *et al.*, 1991). The preparation and purification of antibody is described in *Chapter 2*.

Enzyme preparation: Liver cell extract partially purified by blue A agarose chromatography, to recover 4-sulfatase enriched fraction (Gibson *et al.*, 1987).

Bicarbonate buffer: 0.1 M $NaHCO_3$ pH 8.5

Buffer A: 0.02 mol l^{-1} Tris/HCl, pH 7.0, containing 0.25 mol l^{-1} NaCl

Elution buffer: 0.5 M sodium citrate buffer, pH 4.0 containing 2.0 M NaCl, 10% (v/v) glycerol and 0.02% NaN_3

Protocol

1. Prepare approximately 40 mg of purified monoclonal antibody (see *Chapter 2*).
2. Attach the monoclonal antibody to a solid support (e.g. Affi-Gel 10, BioRad) according to the manufacturer's instructions. Wash 10 ml of Affi-Gel 10 matrix in 3 × 50 ml of ice cold water (rapid washes and minimal aeration of the matrix to avoid oxidation of the succinimide linkages). Add 40 mg of monoclonal antibody in 0.1 M $NaHCO_3$, pH 8.5 to 10 ml of the washed Affi-Gel 10 matrix and incubate with continuous rotation for at least 2 hours at 20°C (4–8 mg of antibody per mL of matrix is ideal). Incubate the matrix and antibody at 4°C overnight, then wash the matrix thoroughly with at least 50 column volumes of buffer A (0.02 mol l^{-1} Tris/HCl, pH 7.0, containing 0.25 mol l^{-1} NaCl, to remove unbound antibody (Buffer A is also a source of amine groups, which will react with and inactivate any remaining active succinimide linkages on the matrix).
3. Pour the monoclonal antibody attached Affi-Gel matrix into a column (~ 20 cm × 1 cm). The entire purification procedure is generally carried out at 4°C. A 5 ml^{-1} pre-column of Affi-Gel 10 washed with buffer A is used to prevent particulates and lipid in samples from entering the affinity column and to remove nonspecific proteins which interact with the matrix.
4. Wash the Affi-Gel 10 antibody matrix column with 20 ml of buffer A prior to use, to remove any free protein, to equilibrate the column and to establish a stable flow rate (0.5–1.0 ml min^{-1}). Add the sample (preferably 10 ml or less

at ≥ 1 mg ml^{-1} total protein, in buffer A) at 0.1–0.5 ml min^{-1} to allow interaction with the antibody matrix. For low affinity antibodies recycling of the load protein may be required for optimal binding, or alternatively the column can be clamped off, and incubated with the loaded sample.

5. Wash the column with at least 10–20 column volumes of buffer A to remove unbound protein. Collect 1–5 ml fractions and assay for the protein of interest, to assess leaching from the matrix and for total protein, to ensure unbound material has been washed off.
6. Add 50 ml of 0.5 M sodium citrate elution buffer, pH 4.0 containing 2.0 M NaCl, 10% (v/v) glycerol and 0.02% NaN_3 to the column at a flow rate of 20 ml h^{-1} (i.e. low pH and high salt elution strategy used for lysosomal proteins). Fractions are assayed, pooled for activity and may then be concentrated and assessed for purity if required (typically homogenous following this procedure: see *Figure 4.6*).

Notes

Affinity chromatography of a protein from a complex mixture (e.g. tissue extract) often requires a preliminary purification step, to reduce either lipid or protein content in the sample, allowing efficient interaction of the key protein with the affinity matrix. The nature of the monoclonal antibody used is also important, as low affinity antibodies will result in protein leaching off the affinity matrix during the purification/wash procedures and very high affinity monoclonal antibodies may prevent easy elution from the affinity matrix.

Different binding and wash conditions can be employed to improve the efficacy of affinity chromatography. Increasing ionic strength (e.g. 0.25 M up to 1.0 M NaCl) can be employed to remove nonspecific binding proteins during the wash procedure. However this approach is limited by the affinity of the monoclonal antibody used for affinity chromatography. High affinity antibodies will allow immuno-affinity chromatography in 1.0 M NaCl, whereas low affinity antibodies may have limited binding even in 0.25 M NaCl. Detergents may also improve the specificity of the chromatography steps. This approach depends on the hydrophobicity of the antigenic determinant bound by the monoclonal antibody and the disruptive effect of the detergent on this interaction.

Elution conditions should favor antigen release but maintain the conformation and activity of the protein to be eluted. Elution strategies must be optimized for each individual antibody/antigen combination. Either low or high pH elution are effective, especially in conjunction with high ionic strength, subject to stability of the protein of interest. Chaotropic agents also are effective, including 8 mol l^{-1} urea, 6 mol l^{-1} guanidine hydrochloride and 6 mol l^{-1} sodium thiocyanate, although these reagents all tend to denature proteins.

Protocol 4.2

Western blotting

Materials

Purified protein: α-L-iduronidase for this example

SDS PAGE: Polyacrylamide gel electrophoresis apparatus and power pack (e.g. BioRad)

Transfer membrane: nitrocellulose membrane or other equivalent (BioRad).

Electoblotting apparatus with power pack (e.g. Hoefer)

Protocol

1. Electrophorese the preparation containing the protein of interest (in this case purified lysosomal protein α-L-iduronidase) in a 10% polyacrylamide gel (Laemmli, 1970) and incorporate the gel in an electroblotting apparatus.
2. Presoak nitrocellulose membrane in buffer A (0.02 mol l^{-1} Tris/HCl, pH 7.0, containing 0.25 mol l^{-1} NaCl), then place it in direct contact with the polyacrylamide gel.
3. 'Sandwich' the gel and the nitrocellulose between wetted sheets of absorbent filter paper and holding pads, then place it in the holding cassette.
4. Place the cassette in the blotting apparatus in buffer C (12.12 g Tris base, 58 g glycine-HCl, 800 ml of methanol, made up to 4 litres in water and adjusted to pH 8.4).
5. Electrophorese towards the anode at 70 V and 800 mA for 60 min using a cooling coil to prevent overheating.
6. After transfer, either prepare the nitrocellulose for immunostaining or remove and wash in buffer A containing 1% w/v Tween 20 for 10 min, then stain for protein by incubation in indian ink solution until developed (200 μl ink in 100 ml of buffer A containing 1% w/v Tween 20). Destain the membrane by rinsing in distilled water.
7. For immunostaining incubate the membrane overnight at 4°C, in buffer B (0.02 mol l^{-1} Tris/HCl, pH 7.0, containing 0.25 mol l^{-1} NaCl and 1% w/v ovalbumin or milk protein), to block nonspecific reactive sites on the membrane.
8. Rinse the membrane in buffer A and incubate with monoclonal antibody culture supernatant (Id1A, a specific monoclonal antibody for human lysosomal enzyme α-L-iduronidase: approximately 10 mg ml^{-1} specific antibody) for at least 4 hours at 20°C.
9. Wash the membrane 3 times in 100 ml of buffer A (10 min for each at 20°C on an orbital shaker), to remove unbound antibody.

10. Incubate the membrane with a 1/200 dilution (in buffer B) of peroxidase labeled sheep anti-mouse immunoglobulin for 1 h at 20°C (sufficient volume to completely immerse the membrane).
11. Wash the membrane three times in 100 ml of buffer A (10 min for each wash at 20°C on an orbital shaker), to remove unbound antibody.
12. Submerge the membrane in 100 ml of buffer A and develop by the addition of 50 ml of 4-chloro-1-naphthol color development reagent (as described by the manufacturer: BioRad).

Note

It is possible to achieve more sensitive immunodetection by chemiluminescence, which effectively amplifies the peroxidase detection step. Antibody detection by enhanced chemiluminescence is available in kit form and is used according to the manufacturer's instructions (NEN Research Products). This normally allows an extension of the sensitivity of protein detection from the ng range to the pg range, depending on the nature and affinity of the primary antibody.

Protocol 4.3

Radiolabel-immunoprecipitation protocol

Materials

[^{35}S]-Cysteine and [^{35}S]-methionine protein labeling mix (1175 Ci mmol^{-1}, NEN Research Products)

75 cm^2 culture flasks, Costar, NY, USA

Cysteine and methionine free Dulbecco's Modified Eagle Medium (Life Sciences)

Dialyzed fetal calf serum

Ham's F-12 medium (GIBCO BRL)

Lysis buffer (10 mM Tris-HCl pH 7.0, 0.15 M NaCl, 4 mM EDTA, 1% (v/v) NP40 plus the protease inhibitors 0.2 mM phenylmethylsulfonyl fluoride, 1 mM pepstatin A, 1 mM leupeptin)

Protein A-Sepharose (Pharmacia)

Amplify (fluor for detection of radioactivity; Amersham International, UK)

Protocol

1. Preincubate cells in 5 ml of cysteine and methionine free Dulbecco's Modified Eagle Medium containing 10% (v/v) dialyzed fetal calf serum, for 60 min and then add 0.3 mCi of [^{35}S]-cysteine and [^{35}S]-methionine protein labeling mix for 5 min–2 h at 37°C.
2. Wash the cells three times with 5 ml of phosphate-buffered saline (PBS) and then either harvest, or chase by adding 5 ml of fresh Ham' s F-12 medium without label, before harvesting.
3. Resuspend the harvested cell pellets in 100 ml of lysis buffer at 4°C.
4. Prepare cell lysates by freeze-thawing the cell pellets six times, then centrifuge out any residual cell debris (12 000 **g** for 5 min at 4°C) and collect the supernatant. Recover the protein in the media from radiolabeled cells (i.e. secreted proteins) by adding 0.3 g ml^{-1} ammonium sulfate overnight at 4°C. Centrifuge (1 000 **g** for 10 min at 4°C) and resuspend the pellets in 1 ml of H_2O, then dialyse twice against 1 liter of 0.25 M NaCl, 0.02 M Tris-HCl pH 7.0 at 4°C .
5. For pre-immunoprecipitation (clearing step) couple a nonspecific antibody to protein A-Sepharose by mixing 1 mg of antibody with 1 ml of packed protein A-Sepharose overnight on a rotator. Centrifuge the protein A-Sepharose-antibody (800 **g** for 1 min) and wash three times with 10 ml 0.25 M NaCl, 0.02 M Tris-HCl pH 7.0. Adjust the extracts to 1 ml in lysis buffer then incubate with 100 ml of the antibody-protein A-Sepharose for at least four hours at 4°C. The supernatants are then recovered by centrifugation (800 **g** for 1 min).

6. Immunoprecipitate the protein of interest as for step 5, except using a specific antibody (attached to fresh protein A Sepharose). After an overnight incubation at 4°C the antigen-antibody protein A-Sepharose is recovered by centrifugation and washed ten times with 10 ml 0.25 M NaCl, 0.02 M Tris-HCl pH 7.0.

7. Dissociate the radiolabeled proteins from the antibody-protein A Sepharose by boiling in reducing SDS-PAGE loading buffer for 5 min, then separate using 10% SDS-PAGE. The gel is recovered and then incubated with the fluor Amplify, for visualization by autoradiography.

The Basics

Chapter 5

Applications of monoclonal antibodies in microbiology

T Kok, P Li, and I Gardner

1. Introduction

Antibodies are useful research tools in the analysis of structure and function of microorganisms, and have become powerful reagents in the diagnosis of infection. Antibody-based specific identification, detection and separation of microorganisms (including viruses) and their antigens form the basis of an array of techniques indispensable to basic research in microbiology, and used increasingly in diagnosis. These techniques include immunoassay, immunostaining for microscopic examination, immunoprecipitation, immunoblotting and separation or purification methods based on immunoaffinity.

The relative advantages of monoclonal and polyclonal antibodies, described in *Chapter 1*, are particularly relevant in microbiology. Diagnosis of bacterial or viral infection needs to be consistent over time, favoring monoclonal antibodies. To understand the pathogenesis of an infection and to design drugs which may inhibit infection, it is vital to have a proper knowledge of the structure of the key molecules involved in the infection process, for example, the surface molecules of a virus which interact with the host cell receptor and mediate viral infection. A homogenous population of epitope specific monoclonal antibody molecules (but not the mixed molecules from a polyclonal antiserum) can be used as a 'structural probe' to stabilize the antigen by forming an antigen–antibody complex that can be crystallized for structural studies. The resolution of the structure of the viral surface envelope glycoprotein gp120 of human immunodeficiency virus (HIV) is a recent example.

Monoclonal antibodies to a large variety of infectious agents are available from commercial sources, from research laboratories on an exchange basis, or produced within the laboratory. In diagnostic infectious disease laboratories, the use of monoclonal antibody offers an efficient means of subtyping viruses (for example herpes simplex virus type I & II).

The highly specific nature of monoclonal antibodies may limit their application. In particular, strain differences may lead to failure of a monoclonal antibody to recognize an organism. Immunoprecipitation or immunoblotting (*Chapter 4*), and the antigen capture part of an enzyme immunoassay can often be better performed by using good quality polyclonal antibodies, because most of the immuno-dominant epitopes of the antigen will be recognized by good quality polyclonal antibodies, while a monoclonal antibody at most can only recognize one of the dominant epitopes. A pool of monoclonal antibodies could be used to cover all the epitopes, but in practise it is easier to use polyclonal antibodies. In diagnostic microbiology, it is common practice to use both polyclonal antibodies and monoclonal antibodies in a single test (see below).

The topics discussed in this chapter involve the applications of monoclonal antibodies in diagnostic and experimental microbiology. Examples of applications with bacteria, viruses, chlamydia and mycoplasma are included. The rationales and advantages in using monoclonal antibodies are illustrated, and particular issues specific to diagnostic microbiology and virology are discussed.

2. Diagnosing infection

The diagnosis of infectious disease is one of the major disciplines in pathology. The means by which a given infection is identified depends on a variety of factors. In general terms infectious organisms are one of four types – bacteria, viruses, fungi, or parasites. There are some basic factors that influence the ease with which these types of infection are diagnosed. For example, bacteria, fungi, and parasites are of sufficient size to be seen under the microscope whereas viruses are too small. Most bacteria can be readily grown from clinical material, as can some viruses and fungi, but parasites generally can not be grown.

The traditional diagnosis of infection required that the organism be seen in or grown from clinical material. This is frequently not possible with adequate sensitivity, for example because the available specimen material contains low numbers of organisms, the organisms are present transiently, a high level of skill is required for microscopic detection, or because of poor viability of the organism and difficulties in culturing the organism. Commensal organisms ('normal flora') can often confuse diagnosis.

Advances have been made in the detection of microorganisms in clinical material. When the organism cannot readily be grown from clinical material, the ability to detect components of the organism, as opposed to whole, viable organism, has led to significant improvement in sensitivity. This sensitivity can also be a problem, for example in latent viral infections where sensitive molecular detection methods can detect minute amounts of virus that do not necessarily represent a reactivation of disease. Care must also be taken in interpreting the detection of microbial antigen or nucleic acid in post-treatment investigation of infection. Sensitive methods may detect small amounts of residual microbial material and give the false impression that therapy has been unsuccessful. In these circumstances detection of live organisms by culture is preferable.

Antigen detection assays initially utilized polyclonal antibodies, usually bound to a solid matrix, to capture the microbial antigens of interest, but increasingly have converted to the use of monoclonal antibodies for the capture step because of their specificity. Cross-reactivity between microorganisms, especially bacteria, is a common problem in antibody-based techniques. Certain bacterial components are common to many different species, and may be similar in structure. An example is bacterial lipopolysaccharide (LPS), which is also highly immunogenic. Polyclonal antisera raised to crude bacterial preparations would be expected to demonstrate a high degree of reactivity to LPS, and in turn may be cross-reactive to a number of bacterial species.

Monoclonal antibodies can mitigate this problem in several ways. Purified antigens can be produced from crude preparations of microorganisms by affinity purification using monoclonal antibodies, and then used to produce monospecific polyclonal antibodies. Alternatively the defined monoclonal antibodies themselves may be used for antigen-capture. However, if the capture antibody reacts with an epitope common to the antigen of interest and other microorganisms, cross-reactivity will still be a problem. In this situation, a monoclonal capture antibody that reacts with an epitope that is highly specific may be the solution. Alternatively, a degree of cross-reactivity in the capture reagent is acceptable, as long as the detection reagent is highly specific.

2.1 Detecting antigen or antibody?

These examples demonstrate that it is sometimes inappropriate to assign diagnostic significance to the presence of an organism or one of its components. Relevant clinical information must be considered. The detection of antibodies in patient sera may be useful under these circumstances. The measurement of the patient's antibody response to the organism, serological diagnosis, is a major part of a diagnostic infectious diseases laboratory. This is a particularly important method in the diagnosis of viral infection as culture and detection methods are less widely available for viruses than they are for bacteria.

The amount or type of antibody can indicate how recently the infection occurred. Originally, this required two separate serum samples and the demonstration of a 'diagnostic' rise in antibody titer over a period of 7–14 days. The final diagnosis was not available until well after the infection had peaked, and often when natural recovery had occurred. The development of isotype-specific antibody assays, primarily using enzyme-linked immunosorbent assay (ELISA), allows the measurement of the antibody isotypes associated with primary immune responses (IgM and IgA) and enables the serological diagnosis of acute infection to be made on a single serum sample.

Serology has a number of practical advantages over methods that detect organisms or their components directly. The techniques used are relatively straightforward and do not require sophisticated equipment or a high degree of technical expertise, the specimen required (normally serum) has often been taken for other purposes, and the result can be available within a few hours. There are however several factors that need to be taken into consideration in interpreting serological results. Antibody responses are inherently variable. Variation may occur in the time of development of antibody, the classes of antibody produced and the range of antibody specificities generated. This latter point is important where relatively crude antigen preparations are used and the antibody measured is the sum of a number of antibody specificities. This can lead to problems of cross-reactivity where some highly antigenic components are similar between different species of organism. Some of these difficulties can be overcome by using purified or recombinant antigens.

Interpretation of serological results requires a high level of training and experience. As well as the issues raised above there are a large number of 'false' reactions that can occur. The actual mechanism of these is not well understood, but certain infections appear to generate a polyclonal stimulation that leads to transient nonspecific antibody responses, particularly IgM responses. While the herpesviruses (especially Epstein-Barr Virus and Cytomegalovirus) are notorious for this, a wide range of other organisms including Parvovirus B19, Hepatitis A virus, *Coxiella burnetii*, and Ross River virus can also show this phenomenon.

In the end the decision of whether to detect the organism directly or use serological methods is dependent on many factors including the expertise in the laboratory, the nature of the organism and the availability of the specimen.

3. Viruses

Viruses are normally smaller than bacteria and do not have ribosomes, mitochondria and other specialized organelles. Consequently, viruses are completely dependent on their host cell for protein synthesis and energy production and unable to grow in nonliving media. Viruses replicate only within host cells. The genetic material of a virus is either DNA or RNA. Bacteria, plants, and animals all play hosts to different viruses. As intracellular parasites, viruses are well known for their ability to cause diseases in humans as well as in animals and plants.

Viral diseases in humans range from mild infections such as the common cold to severe conditions such as acquired immune deficiency syndrome (AIDS, caused by human immunodeficiency viruses, HIV). Mild virus infections are normally self-limiting, where the host immune system responds to the viral infection by mobilizing host cellular (cytotoxic T cells and other killer cells) and humoral (antibody) defences, and suppresses the replication and dissemination of the virus. If the host immune system fails to suppress viral replication and dissemination, as in the case of HIV infection, unchecked viral growth in the body eventually leads to life-threatening conditions. Normally, the dose of infectious virus that initiates infection is very small. It is the ability of the virus to replicate in the host and interactions between the replicating virus and the host that define the pathogenesis of viral infection. A key concept in understanding how viruses infect cells, express their genes and multiply is the viral replication cycle. The accumulation and dissemination of the virus in the host is a result of many such cycles.

Although different viruses employ vastly different replication strategies, there exist three general stages which are common to all viral infections. In the initiation stage, the invading viral particle binds to and penetrates susceptible host cell populations. This stage is of interest to experimental virologists, who use monoclonal antibodies to study the cellular receptor(s) for the virus, the viral ligand (viral surface molecule which binds to the receptor(s)) and the receptor ligand interactions (see below). The second stage is the replication and expression of viral genome. Both experimental and diagnostic virologists are interested in this stage of viral replication. The former may wish to understand the biochemical details of the viral replication strategy and the latter may wish to detect the amplified viral components. Some of the 'early' viral antigens are only expressed in infected cells and not in progeny virus particles and this may allow rapid detection of a virus by immunostaining of the infected cells. (See below, detection of human cytomegalovirus early antigens.) Monoclonal antibodies to these viral antigens are also very important tools for research scientists. The third stage of viral replication involves the assembly, release, and maturation of progeny virus particles. There are important biochemical and molecular details to be studied here for experimental virologists. The released progeny virus particles, containing mature viral structural proteins, are important to diagnostic virologists. Monoclonal antibodies to viral structural proteins are routinely used in many viral diagnostic tests (e.g. HIV p24 tests).

3.1 Experimental virology: monoclonal antibodies as reagents

In this section we describe two examples of application of monoclonal antibodies as reagents in our difficult and unprecedented fight against the human immunodeficiency virus, HIV. This virus has already infected over 40 million and killed more than 11 million people in less than twenty years and is relentlessly extending its reach. Revised estimates (June, 1998) of the spread of HIV indicated that 16 000 people worldwide were being infected every day. In the worst hit countries in sub-Saharan Africa, more than one in eight adults are infected with HIV. The currently available antiretroviral drugs are too expensive to have any real impact in these countries. It is widely believed that, in addition to safe-sex education, the only hope to fundamentally alter the HIV/AIDS epidemic in such countries, is the development of an effective vaccine.

One key target for a vaccine is the viral surface envelope protein gp120, which interacts with the CD4 receptor and a co-receptor on the surface of target cells, to allow the virus to enter the cells and replicate. Detailed structural knowledge about gp120 is important, but its heavily glycosylated structure makes it difficult to crystallize for structural analysis. The CD4 receptor for HIV was crystallized in 1990. It took another eight years to trim the gp120 and grow a crystal containing gp120 for crystallographic analysis, and this was achieved with the help of a monoclonal antibody. The 17b antibody is a broadly neutralizing human monoclonal antibody isolated from the blood of an HIV-infected patient. 17b binds to a CD4 induced gp120 epitope that overlaps the β-chemokine coreceptor binding site. As a result, 17b binds to gp120 tightly only when gp120 is already bound to CD4. The gp120-CD4-17b complex is sufficiently regular to form crystals up to 50 micrometres in diameter – a size just adequate for x-ray crystallography to produce much needed structural information about gp120. This information, published in mid 1998, has already stimulated renewed enthusiasm in HIV vaccine research. Similarly, specific monoclonal antibodies have been used in basic research of surface antigens of other viruses.

Another recent development in HIV/AIDS research is the more detailed understanding of HIV pathogenesis, in particular, the persistent/latent reservoir of HIV in patients. Combination anti-retroviral drugs have made a big difference to the life of millions of HIV infected people in the developed countries. With continued combination drug therapy viral growth is effectively suppressed to very low levels. However, once combination therapy is discontinued, even after years of continuous therapy, HIV will bounce back. To identify the latent/persistent HIV reservoir which enables HIV to survive normal host immune responses in addition to years of highly active antiretroviral therapy, scientists have used an array of murine monoclonal antibodies directed against different human cell surface antigens to separate different cell types in different activation stages, using techniques described in *Chapter 6*. These studies demonstrated that resting CD4 T-cells with a phenotype characteristic of memory cells are most likely to be the long-term latent HIV reservoir. This is important, because new strategies are now being developed to induce this group of latent virus-carrying cells into a more activated state, since HIV-infected activated cells are killed by the combination of continued drug treatment and host immune responses.

3.2 Viral diagnosis: choice of test formats

The usefulness of monoclonal antibody in viral diagnosis may be influenced by the choice of test format. The two commonly used types of assay are the immunofluorescence (IF) and ELISA. Antigen capture ELISA for virus or viral antigen are similar to the antigen capture ELISA described in *Chapter 4*.

The problem of the monoclonal antibody not recognizing a different strain may be overcome by using a cocktail of monoclonal antibodies or by selecting a monoclonal antibody directed towards a conserved antigenic epitope. Alternatively, this arrangement can be used to subtype, for example, herpes simplex virus (HSV) 1 & 2 in clinical samples. The polyclonal rabbit antibody is used as the common capture reagent and the samples tested in two separate microwells with monoclonal antibody to HSV type 1 or 2 as the detector.

Alternatively, monoclonal antibodies can be used to detect specific virus either directly in cells from clinical samples or in virus-infected cell cultures stained with immunofluorescence reagents (*Figures 5.1* and *5.2*). Some laboratories use an immunoperoxidase staining method. There is minimal difference in sensitivity between these two staining methods except that fluorescence may offer increased contrast and hence facilitate observation.

3.3 Detection of class specific antiviral immunoglobulins

The presence of an IgM class specific response to a virus is a marker of current or recent infection. IgG specific antibodies are usually elicited shortly after the IgM response. In some types of re-infections, there is no IgM response but instead IgG specific antibodies are produced. With the detection of class specific (e.g., IgG or IgM) human antiviral immunoglobulins, a commonly used format is to coat a solid support with virus-infected cells. This is then followed by reaction with the test serum and detection with the specific anti-

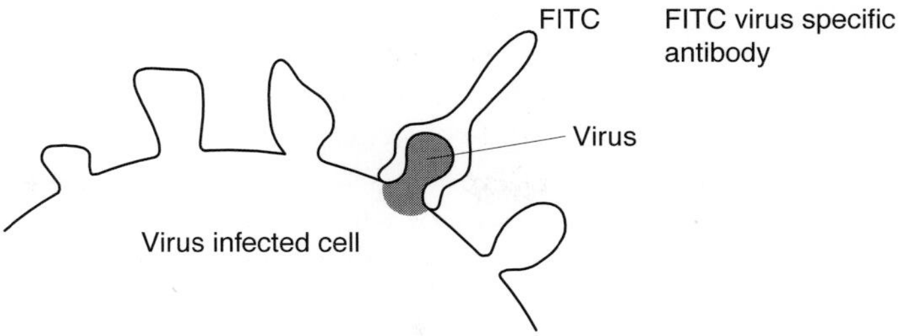

Figure 5.1

Direct immunofluorescence test for detection of virus.

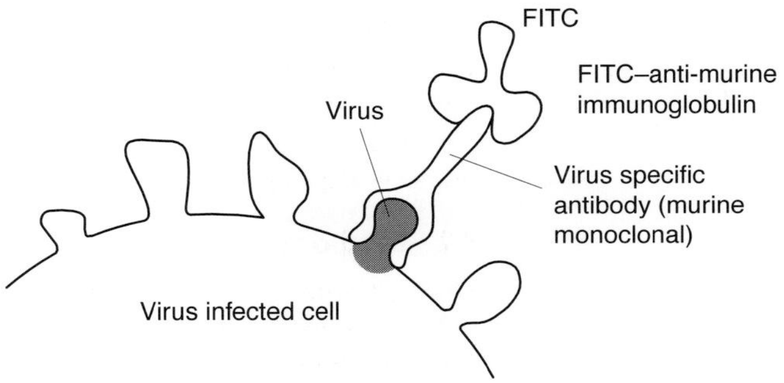

Figure 5.2

Indirect immunofluorescence test for detection of virus.

human γ or μ chain (the heavy chains of IgG and anti IgM respectively). This type of assay may be affected by rheumatoid factors in test sera which can lead to spurious interpretation of results. Rheumatoid factors are auto-antibodies (usually of IgM class) produced against the host's own IgG or other subclasses of immunoglobulins. The use of a heavy chain capture assay (see *Figure 5.3*) has been observed to reduce the interference by rheumatoid factors (the mechanism for this reduced interference has not been characterized). The heavy chain capture antibody is coated in a microwell and is reacted with the test serum. Virus or virus-infected cells are then added which would react with the 'captured' test serum (depending on the anti-heavy chain immunoglobulin used). An enzyme-labelled monoclonal antibody to the virus is then added followed by subsequent reaction with the chromogenic substrate system.

3.4 Detection of cytomegalovirus early antigens

Human cytomegalovirus (CMV) is a member of the Herpesviridae family. The double-stranded DNA genome of CMV is 230 kilobases and has the typical herpes viral sequence organization with a long terminal repeat region at one end and a short terminal repeat at the opposite end. The virus has a diameter that varies from 150–250 nm with an envelope surrounding

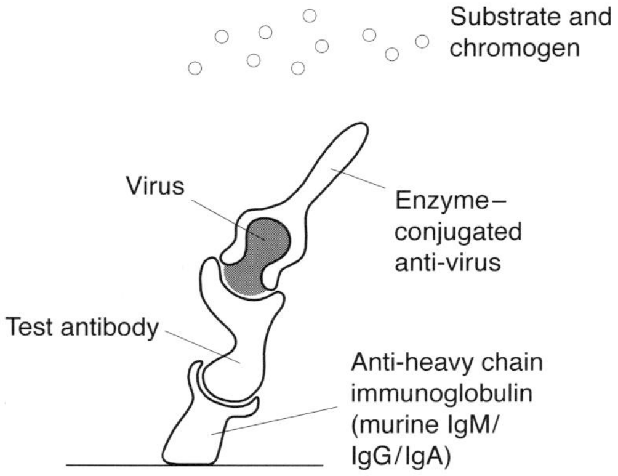

Figure 5.3

Anti-IgM, G, or A capture ELISA for detection of particular classes of anti-viral antibodies.

the nucleocapsid. The chief characteristic of CMV infection, like other herpes viruses, is its persistence in the host. During an opportunistic condition, the latent virus is activated and followed by manifestation of the clinical syndrome. Unlike herpes simplex viruses which remain latent in neurons, CMV latency is maintained in T-lymphocytes or monocytes/macrophages. This virus can be secreted through the urogenital tract and salivary glands. CMV infection occurs in all age groups and in particular the immunosuppressed/deficient patients. In neonates, this virus can cause congenital hepatic, central nervous system or ocular infections and in AIDS patients CMV retinitis is a common syndrome.

In the laboratory, CMV can be isolated only in human fibroblast cells as this virus has a specific host requirement. Due to the slow growth of CMV in cell cultures, which may take up to four weeks to yield cytopathic changes, virus is detected by staining for the immediate early or early viral antigens within 2 days post inoculation. This method is sometimes referred to as 'shell vial' or 'rapid culture' where the specimen is centrifuged at 100 **g** for 1 h onto the fibroblast cell layer. The immediate early or early antigens are detected with monoclonal specific antibodies by fluorescence or peroxidase staining (*Figure 5.4*). A more rapid test with monoclonal antibody to the immediate early antigen may be achieved by staining of peripheral polymorphonuclear leucocytes. A positive result indicates active viral replication and suggests current CMV infection. This is also referred to as the CMV antigenemia test.

4. Mycoplasma and chlamydia

Mycoplasma belong to the Mycoplasmatacae family which is one of two families within the Mollicutes order, and are neither viruses nor bacteria but are usually regarded as the responsibility of virology diagnostic laboratories. Chlamydiae are usually classified as bacteria, but are often also assigned to virology diagnostic laboratories.

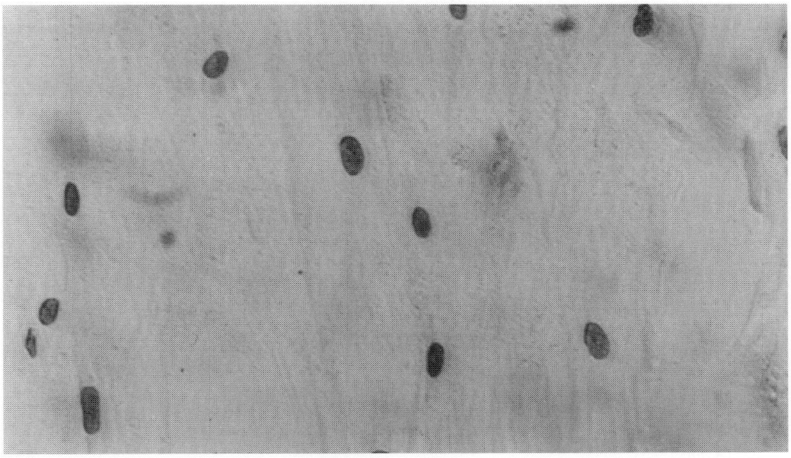

Figure 5.4

Immunoperoxidase staining of cytomegalovirus infected cells. Murine monoclonal antibodies against a cytomegalovirus early antigen were used as detector antibodies.

4.1 Detection of *Mycoplasma pneumoniae*

There are more than forty species of mycoplasmas, of which *Mycoplasma pneumoniae* is a proven pathogen in humans. Recently *M. genitalium* has been associated with human genital as well as respiratory infections. However, *M. pneumoniae* has been the more intensely studied of the human mycoplasmas due to its importance as the causative agent of primary atypical pneumonia. In laboratories, contamination of cell cultures by mycoplasmas is a frequent problem as mycoplasma-infected cells do not show characteristic cytopathology, unlike virus-infected cells, and consequently this can lead to spurious interpretation of experimental results.

Mycoplasma are small, prokaryotic organisms which divide by binary fision. The mycoplasma cell shows a cytoplasmic membrane with a lipid bilayer and contains bacterial-like ribosomes but has no cell wall, unlike bacteria. The average genome size of the single DNA chromosome within the mycoplasma cell is 5×10^8 daltons which is approximately half that of the bacterial genome. Mycoplasmas have a reproductive unit of 125–250 nm, similar to the poxviruses. They may be spherical, filamentous or coccobacillary in form depending on the species and growth conditions. One unique feature of mycoplasmas is their requirement for animal serum in the growth media. The serum provides a source of cholesterol and fatty acids needed for membrane synthesis. Although a number of mycoplasma species are capable of growing on inert media (e.g. agar supplemented with a serum source and yeast extract), in nature they appear in close association with host cells and indeed with *M. pneumoniae* infection the pathology is caused by parasitization of the respiratory ciliated epithelial cells.

Diagnosis has been possible since the 1930s when Liu first used the technically demanding immunofluorescence test on infected chick embryo sections with patients' sera for detection of specific antibodies. For many years diagnosis of this infection relied on detection of specific antibodies in human sera by various immunoassays. It is the rapid detection of this organism or its antigens in respiratory secretions that has required the use of specific antibodies in immunoassays. As *M. pneumoniae* parasitizes on the cell membrane the use of a specific monoclonal antibody in the immunofluorescence test stains the organism on the cell membrane of infected cells. *Figure 5.5a* and *5.5b* show *M. pneumoniae*-infected cells stained with specific monoclonal and polyclonal antibodies in the immunofluorescence test. The use of monoclonal antibody offers the advantage of significantly reduced background staining, which facilitates the subjective observations of specific immunofluorescence.

4.2 Detection of chlamydiae

A major sexually transmitted genital disease in humans is caused by *Chlamydia trachomatis*. This pathogen, which also causes trachoma/inclusion conjunctivitis and neonatal respiratory infection, is one of three chlamydial species in the single Chlamydia genus. The life cycle of the chlamydial organisms involves two major forms – the reticulate body (RB) and the elementary body (EB). The latter is derived from the reticulate body which is non-infective. The RB contains predominantly ribosomal RNA and consists of an outer bilayered membrane surrounding a cytoplasmic membrane. They are found within the cell cytoplasm. In contrast, the EB, which contains the closed circular DNA genome of ~ 1000 kilobase pairs, is the infective form and is found both intracellularly and released during cell lysis. The chlamydial organisms share a genus specific lipopolysaccharide (LPS). The heat-stable LPS is used in diagnostic immunofluorescence tests or enzyme immunoassays with monoclonal specific antibodies (*Figure 5.6*).

The use of the micro-immunofluorescent (MIF) test has enabled the specific serotyping of *C. trachomatis* isolates. Chlamydial EB or isolates are spotted and fixed onto microscope slides. These are then reacted with the specific monoclonal antibody for serotype identification. With the use of specific monoclonal antibodies in the MIF test, *C. trachomatis* isolates can be classified into those that are usually associated with ocular infections (trachoma/conjunctivitis) – serotypes A, B, and C and those associated with human genital infections, which belong to serotypes D to K.

5. Applications in bacteriology

The most common types of infections that are diagnosed in the laboratory are due to bacteria. The isolation of bacteria from clinical specimens and the subsequent determination of antibiotic sensitivities of the isolate are the major roles of most diagnostic microbiology laboratories. The growth of bacterial isolates on a range of selective media and the species identification by a range of techniques is well developed. This is not however appropriate for all bacterial infections. There are certain species that do not grow well on laboratory media and some, notably obligate intracellular organisms, do not grow at all. Others, such as mycobacteria and some anaerobic species,

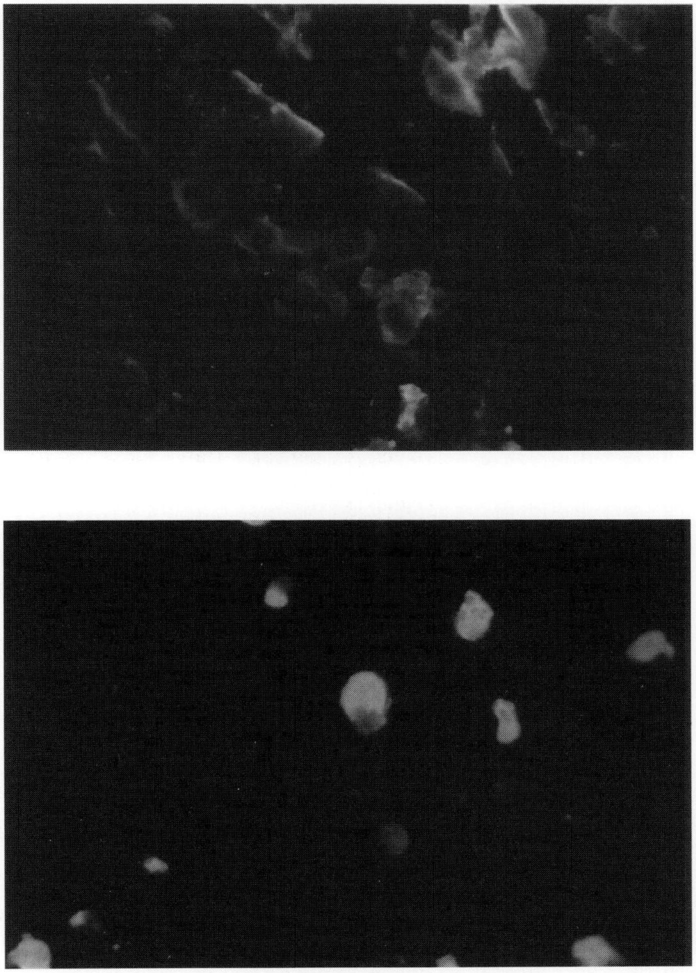

(A)

(B)

Figure 5.5

Immunofluorescence staining of Mycoplasma pneumoniae *infected cells. Rabbit polyclonal antibodies (A) or murine monoclonal antibodies (B) were used as detector antibodies. The reduced background staining in (B) is important in avoiding ambiguous diagnosis.*

take a long time to grow to a point where they can be positively identified by conventional means.

Bacterial infections are normally treatable with antibiotics, and it is important to establish the identity of the infecting bacterium as soon as possible in order to begin appropriate therapy. In a number of cases where growth and identification of bacteria are not adequate, rapid methods have been developed to detect bacterial antigens. This is especially important for potentially serious bacterial infections in critical sites, such as the central nervous system.

The assays originally developed for rapid diagnosis of bacterial antigens used polyclonal antibodies raised in animals such as rabbits. These

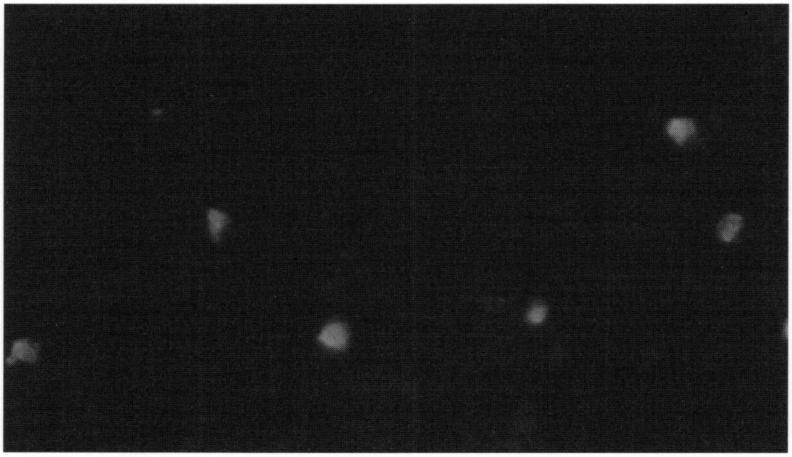

Figure 5.6

Immunofluorescence staining of Chlamydia trachomatis. *Murine monoclonal antibodies against LPS were used as detector antibodies.*

antibodies were usually efficient at binding to bacterial antigens because of their avidity and affinity, but, as discussed earlier, polyclonal reagents are less specific and less reproducible than monoclonal antibodies. In turn, monoclonal antibodies may suffer from cross-reactivity, low affinity or low sensitivity. These problems can often be overcome in the selection process. Hybridoma technology generates a large number of monoclonal antibody-producing clones, and if the appropriate properties can be built into the initial selection criteria it is easier to find a monoclonal antibody with the desired properties than by screening a selection of monoclonals that already exist. Also, questions of low sensitivity can sometimes be addressed by using a pool of two or more antibodies to increase the sensitivity.

Once the monoclonal antibody with the desired properties has been selected, the advantages over polyclonal antibodies become significant. The major costs for monoclonal antibodies are in the development and selection phase, and once the hybridoma clone is stable, continued production of a defined and stable monoclonal antibody is relatively inexpensive.

5.1 Monoclonal antibodies in diagnosis of bacterial infections

The power and specificity of monoclonal antibodies have been used in a number of ways to enhance the diagnosis of bacterial infections. Apart from the replacement of the original polyclonal antibody-based antigen capture assays, the properties of monoclonal antibodies have been used in a variety of innovative ways to help diagnose infections.

Confirmatory identification of bacterial species

There have been several applications of monoclonal antibodies in the absolute identification of bacterial species. This can be useful when the bacteria are difficult to identify from conventional bacterial culture or when time consuming further testing would be required for definitive diagnosis. There are several commercial monoclonal antibody-based assays available for the confirmation of *Neisseria gonorrhoea*. Presumptive isolates have traditionally required a series of biochemical tests to confirm a diagnosis of gonorrhoea infection. The monoclonal antibodies used have been raised against a range of gonococcal protein Is, and enable the differentiation of *N. gonorrhoea* from other non-sexually transmitted *Neisseria* species using a number of techniques including simple agglutination and a colloidal gold-mediated color development test. An IgM monoclonal antibody specific for *Burkholderia pseudomallei* has been used in a simple agglutination assay for the definitive identification of primary bacterial cultures from suspected cases of melioidosis.

Antigen detection assays

The direct detection of bacterial antigens in clinical specimens is one of the common applications of monoclonal antibodies. In many clinical situations whole viable bacteria may not be present in clinical specimens so that culture is not a diagnostic option. Alternatively the important clinical criterion may be the presence or absence of a bacterial product such as a toxin, and the detection of this product may be the important test to do.

The relevant monoclonal antibody is attached to a solid phase, the specimen allowed to react with the antibody and a detection method used to identify the reaction. This type of assay was originally established using polyclonal antibodies but in many cases, while the sensitivity of the assay was acceptable the specificity was not.

Particle-based assays The simplest form of solid phase assay for antigen detection involves the linking of a specific monoclonal antibody to a particle and observing agglutination. This type of methodology is particularly suited to field applications and produces rapid results.

There are a number of assays for bacterial antigen detection using antibody-coated latex particles, some of which are commercially available. The test for *Neisseria meningitidis* uses a monoclonal antibody and will detect *N. meningitidis* antigens in CSF, serum, urine or blood culture medium in cases of bacterial meningitis (Wellcogen Bacterial Antigen Kit, Murex Diagnostics). Specimen and coated latex particles are mixed on a slide and checked for agglutination compared with control latex particles coated with an irrelevant antibody. This assay is described in *Protocol 5.1*.

There are several kits that detect the O1 antigen of *Vibrio cholerae*. This is particularly useful in epidemics of cholera where large numbers of specimens need to be screened in a short time. The simplest form of the assay utilizes killed *Staphylococcus aureus* cells as particles, coated with a monoclonal antibody to the A factor of *V. cholerae* O1 antigen. Stool filtrate is reacted with the coated particles and monitored for agglutination compared with control *S. aureus* particles coated with mouse IgG. A refinement of this assay uses the same monoclonal antibody linked to colloidal gold. This is reacted with stool filtrate, and complexed antibody is detected with a second antibody producing a red spot in the presence of antigen.

A rapid serotype specific test has been developed for *Salmonella enteritidis*. This test uses latex particles coated with monoclonal antibodies to fimbrial antigens. One antibody detects the SEF fimbriae expressed by both *S. enteritidis* and *S. dublin*, and the other is specific for *S. dublin*. The differential reactivity of the two reagents with Salmonella isolates allows the rapid identification and serotyping of *S. enteritidis*.

The slow growth of mycobacterial species in culture can cause delays in the definitive diagnosis of infection, and there are difficulties in distinguishing *M. tuberculosis* from other mycobacteria. A particle counting immunoassay has been developed for the detection of mycobacterial antigens after short-term culture. Latex particles coated with polyclonal anti-BCG detected mycobacterial antigens several days before an automated culture system, and particles coated with an *M. tuberculosis*-specific monoclonal antibody routinely identified *M. tuberculosis* cultures.

A different application of particle technology has been used in a veterinary setting to detect leptospira in the urine of cows. Leptospira specific monoclonal antibody-coated magnetic particles were reacted with urine to capture leptospiral antigen, and this was detected using a second monoclonal antibody labeled with biotin. The signal was detected in a fluoroimmunoassay using europium-labeled streptavidin. This assay did not offer significantly better sensitivity than conventional culture, but did detect antigen in a number of culture-negative animals as well as giving a more rapid result. In these circumstances it would be prudent to use both techniques for the best results.

Enzyme immunoassays (ELISA) A logical step in the evolution of antigen detection assays is to enhance the sensitivity by signal amplification. While this is obviously desirable from a diagnostic point of view, assays of this type require more sophisticated technology and are effectively restricted to the laboratory, unlike agglutination tests that are suited to application in the field. Antigen detection ELISAs are normally antigen capture assays, as described in *Chapter 4*.

One of the first commonly-used antigen detection ELISAs was for *Chlamydia trachomatis* antigen in genital specimens. There are a number of assays on the market, many of them using a monoclonal antibody or mixtures of monoclonal antibodies. The most common antigen to be detected is the chlamydial lipopolysaccharide (LPS) as this is the most soluble chlamydial antigen. It is also highly immunogenic. Chlamydia ELISA tests are reasonably sensitive, although much less so than the newer molecular assays. One issue with these ELISAs is the relatively low specificity, which is a problem with a sexually-transmitted disease, especially when screening a low-prevalence population. It is necessary to confirm positives using a blocking assay where the specimen is pre-reacted with a known monoclonal antibody to chlamydial LPS. True positives are blocked by this, false positives are not.

Another antigen detection ELISA detects protein antigens of *Mycobacterium tuberculosis* in serum specimens from patients being studied for infertility. This sandwich assay uses a polyclonal antibody to BCG as primary capture antibody and horseradish peroxidase (HRP)-conjugated monoclonal antibody as secondary antibody. The combination of polyclonal antibody to capture antigen and monoclonal antibody to detect captured antigen is often used. It benefits from the sensitivity and avidity of the polyclonal antibody followed by the specificity of the monoclonal antibody, leading to the best possible outcome.

Antigen detection can be particularly important in situations where serological diagnosis is the normal method and where an antibody response has not been detected. A subset of patients with neurological Lyme disease do not make a serological response to *Borrelia burgdorferi*. An antigen detection ELISA using monoclonal antibodies was developed to measure the OspA antigen of *B. burgdorferi* in CSF. This assay detected OspA antigen in CSF in the absence of serum antibody and may be an important adjunct to serology in the diagnosis of neurologic Lyme disease.

Enteric fever as a result of infection with *Salmonella* species is common in some countries. There is a need for rapid and simple tests to diagnose Salmonella infections in these circumstances. A monoclonal antibody-based dot-blot ELISA was developed for measuring Salmonella antigenuria in patients with clinical features of enteric fever. This assay showed good sensitivity and specificity compared with the classical methods of bacterial culture and serology by the Widal test, and was straightforward to perform in developing areas.

Other sandwich ELISAs for bacterial antigens have been developed and show potential for future diagnostic uses. A monoclonal antibody to the lipopolysaccharide of *Moraxella (Branhamella) catarrhalis* was incorporated into an ELISA, and demonstrated the ability to selectively detect soluble LPS from all *M. catarrhalis* species but not from other related and unrelated respiratory bacteria. Another assay utilized monoclonal antibody to *Burkholderia pseudomallei* in a sandwich ELISA to detect antigens in clinical specimens from patients with culture-proven melioidosis. A sandwich ELISA using monoclonal antibodies reactive with components of the flagella of *Salmonella paratyphi*, the agent of paratyphoid fever, successfully detected flagellin antigens in serum samples from patients with acute disease. Each of these assays shows promise in early diagnosis of infection, as conventional means of diagnosis are not straightforward in infections with these bacteria.

Toxin detection There is a definite clinical need to detect the presence of bacterial toxins in certain bacterial infections. The toxins produced by some bacteria have a direct role in the pathogenesis of the infection, and the earlier the identification the sooner appropriate treatment can be instituted and the pathogenic effects of the toxin curtailed. The traditional method of detecting bacterial toxins has been assessing the effects of the toxin on cell culture. This has led to classification of toxins by their effect on cultured cells, e.g. verocytotoxins, which selectively kill Vero cells.

Clostridium difficile infection is the major cause of both antibiotic-associated diarrhoea and pseudomembranous colitis. There are two major toxins produced by this organism, an enterotoxin (toxin A) and a cytotoxin (toxin B). Toxin A is more stable and as both are produced in infection has been chosen as the target for detection assays. There are several commercial assays that detect *C. difficile* toxin A in stool solution supernatant. A sandwich ELISA using polyclonal capture antibody and monoclonal detector antibody is commonly used. This can be found in a conventional 96-well microplate format or in a more convenient immunoassay system (VIDAS, bioMerieux Vitek) where the test is done in a closed cassette and requires no manipulation during the assay.

Other bacterial species are associated with toxins of clinical relevance. *Shigella dysenteriae* produces Shiga toxin, which is the pathogenic factor in Shigella-associated diarrhoea, prevalent in conditions of poor sanitation. A sandwich ELISA using a polyclonal/monoclonal combination was developed for Shiga toxin. This assay successfully detected the toxin in stools of patients with *S. dysenteriae* type 1 infection with a high degree of sensitivity (100 pg). This assay has a high degree of specificity as it did not detect toxin from other Shigella species or the closely related Shiga-like toxin produced by enterohemorrhagic *Escherichia coli* (EHEC).

E. coli toxins are also important clinically. The verocytotoxin-producing *E. coli* (VTEC) pose an important public health issue, and it is important to detect environmental sources of these bacteria. A monoclonal antibody-based sandwich ELISA has been developed to detect *E. coli* verocytotoxins 1 and 2 in feces of animals. This assay could detect toxin produced by less than 1000 toxin-producing *E. coli* per gram of feces after a short period of culture.

Enterotoxigenic *E. coli* (ETEC) produce both heat stable (ST) and heat labile (LT) toxins. ELISAs have been developed to identify *E. coli* isolates producing these clinically important toxins. The assay to identify LT-producing isolates uses the GM1 ganglioside receptor molecule bound to microtiter wells to capture LT, and enzyme labeled polyclonal or monoclonal antibodies as detector antibodies. Measurement of ST-producing isolates uses a competitive binding ELISA. Supernatants from *E. coli* cultures are tested for the ability to inhibit a microplate ELISA system using bound STa-BSA conjugate with a monoclonal antibody to STa.

Microscopic methods

One of the major applications of monoclonal antibodies to diagnosis of bacterial infections has been their use in microscopy. The specificity inherent with monoclonal antibodies can often allow a more detailed understanding of the antigenic nature of organisms and their distribution within tissue than is possible with polyclonal antisera.

Immunohistochemistry Diagnosing the presence of bacterial infection can present some difficulties when the organism is restricted to solid tissue and not normally found in sites that can be readily sampled. In these circumstances the visualization of the organism in tissue sections can be a useful way to confirm infection. Monoclonal antibodies are not always particularly successful at identifying antigenic epitopes in formalin-fixed tissues, which can be restrictive given that the majority of tissue specimens are prepared this way. Strategies have been used to create more 'robust' monoclonal antibodies, including immunization with formalin-fixed material and doing the primary screening on formalin-fixed tissue.

The disease ehrlichosis, caused by infection with *Ehrlichia chaffeensis*, has recently been recognized as a significant problem in certain regions. A monoclonal antibody to *E. chaffeensis* was used to stain sections of human kidney, lung and liver by immunohistology to detect the organism. This antibody is directed at a surface epitope and is highly specific, not reacting with other bacteria including *E. canis*.

Chlamydia pneumoniae is a respiratory infection that causes an atypical pneumonia. Recent studies have associated *C. pneumoniae* infection with atherosclerotic cardiovascular disease, although the mechanism of this association is not known. Attempts have been made to demonstrate the presence of *C. pneumoniae* in atheromatous plaque with varying success. A recent immunohistochemical study used a range of genus- and species-specific chlamydial monoclonal antibodies to identify *C. pneumoniae* in the cardiac blood vessels of patients with arteriosclerosis.

Epidemic louse-borne typhus is a disease caused by infection with the rickettsial species *Rickettsia prowazekii*. Rickettsia are difficult to culture and the routine serology (Weil-Felix) test is relatively nonspecific, relying on a cross reaction with Proteus organisms. Detection of organisms in biopsy tissue is a definitive way of diagnosing the infection. A monoclonal antibody specific for a lipopolysaccharide epitope of *R. prowazekii* was used to detect the organism in formalin-fixed paraffin-embedded tissue by immunohistochemistry. Interestingly, three of the detections were from brains of people who had died over 50 years previously. Thus this approach may be of use in studying archival material as well as providing a relatively rapid diagnosis of typhus.

Direct fluorescent antibody (DFA) test The use of fluorescent labels on antibodies and the visualization of binding under high intensity illumination has become a major technique in the rapid diagnosis of infections. The fluorochrome used most often is fluorescein isothiocyanate (FITC) which is excited by blue light at 490–495 nm and emits a characteristic green fluorescence at 517 nm. Many laboratories have a microscope with incident light fluorescent illumination and the appropriate excitation and barrier filters that can be used for this purpose.

It is important to explain an inconsistency of terminology at this point. In a diagnostic setting the term 'direct fluorescent antibody' refers to the use of an antibody to detect microbial antigen in a clinical specimen. This antibody may be directly conjugated with a fluorochrome (*Figure 5.1*) or it may be used in a two-stage assay with a fluorochrome-labeled second antibody (*Figure 5.2*); both are called 'direct'. In contrast, the term 'indirect fluorescent assay (IFA)' is reserved for assays that measure antibody, where patient serum is reacted with a substrate containing microbial antigen and the presence of specific antibodies in the serum detected by a fluorochrome-labeled antihuman immunoglobulin. The confusion that may arise is the convention in other settings that a two-stage assay using an unlabeled primary antibody followed by a fluorochrome-labeled second antibody is referred to as an 'indirect' assay (see *Chapter 6*).

A well-established diagnostic use for DFA in bacterial infections is in testing for *Chlamydia trachomatis*. Infection of the genital tract with

C. trachomatis is considered to be the leading cause of pelvic inflammatory disease and consequent infertility in females in the Western world. DFA testing allows a rapid and sensitive diagnosis of this infection, which is readily treatable with antibiotics. There are many FITC-labeled monoclonal antibodies on the market that are used to detect chlamydial elementary bodies in clinical specimens, usually genital swabs but occasionally from eye swabs. The monoclonal antibodies are usually of two types – either directed against the chlamydial lipopolysaccharide (LPS) which reacts with all members of the Chlamydia genus, or against the major outer membrane protein (MOMP) of *C. trachomatis*, which is specific for that species. DFA testing for *C. trachomatis* is still used widely, but the evolution of molecular methods for DNA detection and the skill level required will inevitability decrease its diagnostic use.

Recent years have seen the emergence of another member of the chlamydia genus, *C. pneumoniae*, as a major human respiratory pathogen. Unlike *C. trachomatis*, *C. pneumoniae* cannot be detected readily by cell culture, antigen detection or molecular methods. Diagnosis is generally made on serological grounds, but this serology is technically complex (IFA) and the clinical significance not fully understood. It is possible to detect *C. pneumoniae* organisms in respiratory specimens using DFA, although good diagnostic monoclonal antibodies are difficult to obtain. An alternative strategy is to stain the specimen with the genus-specific LPS monoclonal antibody, and if positive stain with the *C. trachomatis*-specific MOMP monoclonal antibody. Positivity against LPS but not MOMP implies but does not confirm the presence of *C. pneumoniae*.

A diverse range of other bacteria can be detected using DFA, and a selection of these applications is presented. A monoclonal antibody to a lipooligosaccharide epitope of *Bordetella pertussis* was used to detect organisms from nasopharyngeal swabs in the investigation of whooping cough. The commercial test for direct detection of *Legionella pneumophila* in respiratory specimens uses an FITC-labeled monoclonal antibody (Genetic Systems). The most specific means of diagnosing syphilis is by direct visualization of *Treponema pallidum* in lesion material, and FITC-labeled monoclonal antibody can be used for this assay. The presence of *Vibrio cholerae* O139 can be detected in 20 minutes in stool specimens with a high degree of sensitivity and the use of a single FITC-labeled monoclonal antibody.

Flow cytometry The detection of fluorescent label can be done by means other than direct examination under a fluorescent microscope. Analysis of labelled cell populations by flow cytometry has a number of significant advantages over routine microscopy, including the ability to set objective criteria for positivity and the capacity to analyze large numbers of particles in a short time (see *Chapter 6* for a detailed discussion of flow cytometry).

Flow cytometry using monoclonal antibodies to detect microorganisms in clinical specimens has never become established as a routine diagnostic tool. There are however a number of applications of flow cytometry of bacteria that have increased understanding of the infective process. One example of this is the study of the capsular polysaccharides of *Staphylococcus aureus* and the role that they play in the interaction with host cells. A monoclonal antibody to the *S. aureus* capsular polysaccharide type 5 was used by flow cytometry to quantitate the amounts of CP5 in a range of *S. aureus* isolates and to relate these amounts to the origin of the isolate and to the cultivation medium.

There have been some applications to direct detection of bacteria from food. A novel system was devised using a combination of an FITC-labeled monoclonal antibody to *Salmonella typhimurium* and a fluorogenic marker for cell viability in a flow cytometry assay system. This system was able to detect levels of viable *S. typhimurium* as low as 100 cells ml^{-1} of specimen, even in the presence of large numbers of organisms of different species or dead organisms. This type of assay has great potential in the food microbiology industry.

5.2 Adjuncts to molecular methods

There has been a major increase in the number of methods that use molecular techniques for diagnosis of microbial infections. In some cases these are effectively replacing the assay methods of the past, including those that use monoclonal antibodies. A prime example of this is the detection of *Chlamydia trachomatis*. The 'gold standard' method was cell culture, with chlamydial inclusions stained by iodine. The development of chlamydial monoclonal antibodies led to their use, FITC-labeled, to stain these inclusions as well as in DFA examination of clinical smears. These same antibodies became the basis for the antigen capture ELISA that provided the first semiautomated assay for large-scale screening. The application of the polymerase chain reaction (PCR) and later the ligase chain reaction (LCR) to the detection of chlamydia has revolutionized this testing, but only for those laboratories able to utilize this relatively sophisticated technology. There is still a large role for monoclonal antibody-based testing in the routine diagnosis of *C. trachomatis* infection.

A number of molecular techniques have evolved that utilize monoclonal antibodies in the preparatory stages. A common example is the use of immunomagnetic separation of the organism of interest prior to the amplification of target DNA by PCR. Coating of specific monoclonal antibody onto magnetic beads allows the capture of relatively small numbers of organisms from a large volume of sample, and permits the 'cleaning-up' of the preparation to remove possible inhibitors of the PCR reaction. This has been done for detection of *Shigella dysenteriae* and *Shigella flexneri* from feces, *Porphyromonas gingivalis* from oral specimens, *Mycobacterium avium* in stool samples from AIDS patients and salmonella species from stool specimens. Apart from these directly clinical applications this combination of technologies could have broad applicability for situations where the target for DNA amplification is present in low numbers in a large volume of potentially inhibitory material.

5.3 Serological diagnosis of bacterial infection

There are times where it is necessary to diagnose or confirm that infection with a certain organism has occurred, and where it is not possible to use direct detection methods to identify the organism. This may be because the appropriate specimen is unavailable or because all traces of the organism have disappeared.

There are many different methods used for the serological diagnosis of bacterial infection. The more traditional methods are simple agglutination tests (such as the Widal for salmonella and the Weil-Felix for rickettsia) and complement fixation. The introduction of more sensitive and specific testing methods such as indirect immunofluorescence (IFA) and microplate ELISA have made serological testing much better, but there are a number of important bacterial infections for which these improved technologies have not been developed. In some cases this deficiency is due to a perceived lack of importance of serological diagnosis for the particular infection, but in other cases there are significant technical problems. This is especially true for ELISA serology where there may be difficulties in obtaining an appropriate antigen preparation to coat onto the solid phase.

In a number of bacterial infections this has been overcome with the help of monoclonal antibodies in an inhibition or blocking ELISA. This method has as its basis a test system with antigen on the solid phase and a known monoclonal antibody to that antigen as the binding antibody. The antigen may be purified or recombinant but may also be a crude extract, as the monoclonal antibody gives the system its specificity. The presence of antibodies in a serum can be determined by the extent to which that serum competes with the monoclonal antibody in binding to the defined antigen, thereby reducing the amount of signal generated by the labeled monoclonal antibody. By its nature the inhibition ELISA uses lower concentrations of serum than direct ELISA, reducing the problem of nonspecific binding.

There are many examples where this type of inhibition ELISA has provided a better measure of serological response than other methods. The diagnosis of typhoid fever due to infection with *Salmonella typhi* has often been made on serological grounds using the Widal test, although this is not particularly sensitive or specific. Sera from typhoid patients show strong reactivity to porins in the bacterial cell wall, but there is broad cross reactivity with porins from other gram-negative bacteria. An inhibition ELISA was established using a test system of specific *S. typhi* porins as antigen and enzyme-conjugated specific monoclonal antibody. The serum antibodies detected by inhibition of this test system were highly specific for proven typhoid fever status and the assay performed significantly better than the Widal assay.

Mycobacterial infections are another group where there are problems of diagnosis. Serological testing has not been established as a routine because of broad cross-reactivity between species. Inhibition ELISA tests for serum antibody have been developed for several mycobacterial species. Serodiagnosis of tuberculosis was established using a test system of soluble extract of *M. tuberculosis* coated onto the solid phase and a specific monoclonal antibody. Similar restrictions exist for the serodiagnosis of leprosy. The inhibition ELISA for specific antibodies to *M. leprae* also used a soluble bacterial extract as antigen, and a monoclonal antibody to the 35 kDa antigen. Antibodies detected by this assay system showed good correlation with mycobacterial load and could be useful in monitoring response to therapy.

The O157-H7 strain of *Escherichia coli* has recently emerged as a significant human pathogen, being involved in a number of conditions including hemolytic uremic syndrome. It is carried in the gastrointestinal tracts of farm animals but shed intermittently, making identification of infected animals difficult. Serological identification of animals carrying O157-H7 would be highly desirable. The O157 antigen shares common elements with the lipopolysaccharide (LPS) of other bacterial species, including *Brucella abortus* and *Yersinia enterocolitica*, so an inhibition ELISA was developed to measure antibodies specific for the O157-H7 of *E. coli*. The assay used *E. coli* O157-H7 LPS as antigen and a monoclonal antibody specific for *E. coli* O157 as competing antibody. This assay showed a high degree of specificity and good sensitivity in cattle, and has considerable promise as a screening assay to detect animals carrying this potentially harmful strain of *E. coli*.

6. Parasitic and fungal infections

Many of the monoclonal antibody-based techniques described in the section on diagnosis of bacterial infection have been applied to the diagnosis of parasitic and fungal infections.

Parasites as a general rule cannot be cultured in the normal laboratory setting, and traditionally their diagnosis has relied on routine microscopy. This requires considerable experience and skill to detect the subtle morphological differences between different species. The development of parasite-specific monoclonal antibodies has allowed a more definitive speciation of parasites in clinical specimens. Examples of parasitic infections where monoclonal antibody DFA has been used on stool specimens include *Giardia lamblia*, *Cryptosporidium parvum*, and *Encephalitozoon intestinalis*.

Extensive use has been made of monoclonal antibody-based antigen capture ELISAs for the detection of circulating parasitic antigens in human serum. These include *Fasciola hepatica*, *Wuchereria bancroftii*, *Toxoplasma gondii*, *Parastrongylus cantonensis*, *Leishmania donovani* and *Angiostrongylus malaysiensis*. Similar assays have been used to detect parasitic antigens in other specimens such as feces (*Entamoeba histolytica*, *Schistosoma japonicum*, *Opisthorcis viverrini*), urine (*Trypanosoma cruzii*, *Onchocerca volvulus*, *Schistosoma mansonii*), and liver cyst aspirate (*Echinococcus granulosus*).

Considerable attention has been given to the diagnosis of malaria, the most significant parasitic disease in the world. Malaria has traditionally been diagnosed by microscopic detection of parasites in blood films, which is time consuming, operator-dependent and relatively insensitive. Rapid antibody-based assays have been developed recently to improve this diagnosis, and a number of these utilize monoclonal antibodies. An IFA test using FITC-labeled monoclonal antibody reactive with *Plasmodium vivax* erythrocytic stage antigen was shown to be effective in the diagnosis of *P. vivax* in blood films. *Plasmodium falciparum* can be detected in whole blood using antigen-capture assays based on a monoclonal antibody to the histidine-rich protein (HRP-II) of *P. falciparum*. These have been adapted to a cartridge format with a colour readout (ParaSight-F, Becton-Dickinson; ICT Malaria P.f., AMRAD). More recently a dipstick test for whole blood has been developed which can detect *P. falciparum* and *P. vivax* in the same sample. This test utilizes a combination of species-specific and genus-specific monoclonal antibodies against the plasmodium intracellular metabolic enzyme pLDH, and the pattern of reactivity determines whether the infection is with *P. falciparum* or *P. vivax* (OptiMAL, Flow Inc.).

Systemic fungal infections are less common than infections with viruses, bacteria and parasites. They are however becoming a significant problem in immuno-compromised patients, and the conventional detection methods of culture and microscopy do not always have adequate sensitivity, specificity and rapidity. A number of monoclonal antibody-based methods have been developed to aid the rapid diagnosis of fungal infections.

Detection of *Cryptococcus neoformans* antigens is a routine laboratory test in AIDS and other immunocompromised patients. These assays use antibody-coated latex particles to detect circulating antigen in serum or CSF in cases of suspected cryptococcal meningoencephalitis. Monoclonal antibodies have replaced the original polyclonal antibodies in the latest versions of this assay. A similar monoclonal antibody-based particle assay is used to detect *Aspergillus galactomannan* antigen in the serum of patients with invasive aspergillosis, and a highly sensitive antigen capture ELISA has also been developed to detect the same antigen. Infection with *Histoplasma capsulatum* is endemic in some areas of the world and may lead to disseminated histoplasmosis if untreated. Serological testing is of little use, and testing for circulating antigen with a sensitive inhibition ELISA using specific monoclonal antibodies shows great promise.

The other major fungal disease that is a significant problem in immunocompromised and AIDS patients is pneumonia due to *Pneumocystis carinii* infection (PCP). The rapid diagnosis of PCP is vital in the clinical setting. Microscopy of silver stained sputum specimens has been the method of choice, but this technique is technically demanding and not particularly sensitive. Monoclonal antibodies to *P. carinii* labeled with FITC have been produced commercially and DFA is now the first line test for sputum specimens in many laboratories.

Monoclonal antibodies have been used extensively in immunohistochemical identification of fungi in suspected fungal infections. Species specific monoclonal antibody against galactomannan of Aspergillus species was successful in detecting Aspergillus in formalin-fixed wax-embedded tissue specimens. A monoclonal antibody against the capsular polysaccharide of *Cryptococcus neoformans* has been used to localize cryptococcal antigens in central nervous system tissue in cases of cryptococcal meningoencephalitis. Monoclonal antibodies to *Paracoccidioides brasiliensis* were able to specifically identify that organism in paraffin-embedded sections of human biopsy material. Invasive *Candida albicans* infection with cutaneous dissemination was rapidly confirmed in a patient by immunohistochemical staining of a skin biopsy using monoclonal antibody to *C. albicans* mannan antigen.

Further reading

White, D.O. and Fenner, F.J. (1994) *Medical Virology*, 4th edn. Academic Press, San Diego, CA.

Lennette, E.H., Halonen, P. and Murphy, F.A. (eds) (1988) *Laboratory diagnosis of infectious diseases. Principles and practice, vol II. Viral, rickettsial and chlamydial diseases*. Springer-Verlag, New York.

Li, P. and Kok, T.W. (1997) Medical Virology, In: *Principles and practice of medical laboratory science* (ed. Leong, A.S.Y.), vol II, pp 81–186. Churchill Livingstone, London.

Herrman, J.E. (1995) Immunoassays for the Diagnosis of Infectious Diseases. In: *Manual of Clinical Microbiology* (eds. Murray, P.R., Baron, E.J., Pfaller, M.A., Tenover, F.C., Yolken, R.H.), 6th edn, pp. 110–122. American Society for Microbiology, Washington.

Isenberg, H.D. (ed.) (1992) *Clinical Microbiology Procedures Handbook*, vol. 2, section 9. American Society for Microbiology, Washington.

Protocol 5.1

Detection of *Neisseria meningitidis* antigen by agglutination of monoclonal antibody-coated latex particles, using the Wellcogen Bacterial Antigen Test Kit as a model (Murex Biotech, Dartford, UK – now a part of Abbott Laboratories, Abbott Park, USA)

Equipment

Disposable reaction cards

Disposable mixing sticks

Disposable droppers

Boiling waterbath

Laboratory centrifuge

Rotator (optional)

Reagents

N. meningitidis B/*E. coli* K1 Test Latex (0.5% suspension in buffer, coated with specific monoclonal antibody)

Control Latex (0.5% suspension in buffer, coated with irrelevant monoclonal antibody)

Polyvalent Positive Control

0.1 M EDTA, pH 7.4

Specimens

Serum, cerebrospinal fluid (CSF) or urine

Blood culture

Protocol Part A – Preparation of specimens

1. CSF and urine samples are heated 5 min in a boiling waterbath, cooled to room temperature and clarified by centrifugation.
2. Serum is diluted with 3 volumes of 0.1 M EDTA, pH 7.4, heated 5 min in a boiling waterbath and clarified by centrifugation.
3. Blood culture (1–2 ml) is centrifuged to pellet the red cells (1000 **g** for 5–10 min) and the supernatant tested. If a nonspecific reaction occurs with the unsensitized particles, the supernatant should be heated, cooled and centrifuged as described above.

Protocol Part B – Test procedure

1. Process the specimen as described above.
2. Shake the latex reagents to suspend the particles.
3. Place 1 drop of each of **test latex** or **control latex** onto a separate circle on a reaction card. Ensure that the dropper bottles are held vertically to dispense an accurate drop.
4. Using a disposable dropper, dispense 1 drop of **test sample** next to each drop of latex.
5. Mix the contents of each circle with a mixing stick and spread to cover the complete area of the circle. Use a separate stick for the test and control circles and discard each stick after use.
6. Rock the card slowly and observe for agglutination for 3 min, holding the card at normal reading distance (25–35 cm) from the eyes. Alternatively, a mechanical rotator may be used for 3 min. The patterns obtained are clear-cut and can be recognized under all lighting conditions (*Figure 5.7*).
7. Discard the used Reagent Card and mixing sticks for safe biohazard disposal.
8. The positive reaction is quality controlled by doing a separate reaction using one drop of the polyvalent control in place of the test sample.

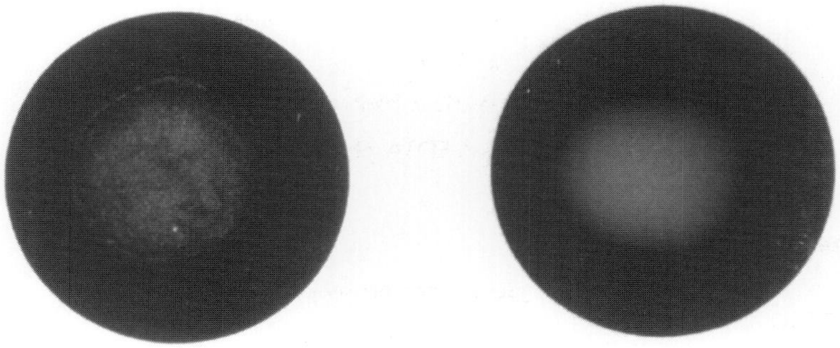

Figure 5.7

Results of latex agglutination assay (see Protocol 5.1*). A positive sample shows agglutination (clumping) while a negative test leaves the latex particles in uniform suspension.*

Reference

Kit Insert from Murex Wellcogen Bacterial Antigen Kit ZL26, Murex Biotech Ltd, Central Road, Temple Hill, Dartford, Kent, DA1 5LR, U.K.

Note

The protocol described here is for a commercial test kit, where antibody-coated particles are provided. It is relatively straightforward to utilize this methodology for the detection of a range of antigens. Proteins, including monoclonal antibodies, adsorb efficiently onto latex and a number of other particles (charcoal, bentonite) at a slightly alkaline pH. Slide or tube agglutination reactions to detect the relevant antigens can be done with a low background protein concentration in the mixture (too much protein prevents agglutination, too little may cause false-positive reactions).

The Basics

Chapter 6

Applications of monoclonal antibodies to the study of cells and tissues

H Zola

1. Introduction

One of the major successes of monoclonal antibodies has been their application to the study of cells and tissues. Monoclonal antibodies have made possible a detailed analysis of the functional molecules on the cell surface, the molecules which mediate the interactions between cells and other cells or between cells and other components of their environment. Once these molecules were identified with monoclonal antibodies, it was possible to clone the genes coding the molecules, which in turn provided new analytical probes and allowed exploration of the control of expression of the molecules. In recent times it has been possible to identify molecules, such as receptors for growth factors, at the messenger RNA level first, without the need for antibodies, but the majority of the cell surface molecules we know were identified initially with monoclonal antibodies.

Whilst the molecular composition of the cell surface is better understood than that of the cell interior, the functional machinery of the cell as a whole is gradually being elucidated, and antibodies provide essential reagents for these studies.

Antibodies have also been particularly useful as markers for different cell types. Whilst many molecules involved in cellular function will be expressed by many different cell types, some components, particularly of the cell membrane, are uniquely required by particular cells for their specific function. For example, immunoglobulin is a defining characteristic of B lymphocytes; hemoglobin of red cells. These molecules serve as markers for their particular cell type, and monoclonal antibodies generally provide the best probe to identify the marker. Once an antibody is available as a marker for a particular cell type, it can be used to identify the cells in tissue, to count cells in tissue or in a suspension, to separate out cells with the help of physical separation procedures which distinguish cells coated with antibody from uncoated cells, or to destroy the cells using a cytotoxic agent linked to the antibody. In many instances antibody against a functional surface molecule can act as an agonist, triggering the cellular function normally mediated through that molecule. In some instances the opposite happens, and the antibody inhibits the function; in either case antibodies can be used as probes for cellular function.

2. The complexity of cells: the human CD antigens illustrate the heterogeneity of cellular composition

We will examine the analysis of human leukocyte membrane antigens, as an example of the analytical power of monoclonal antibodies in cellular studies. Because of their importance in understanding, monitoring and modulating the immune system, this group of antigens has been very extensively studied, largely through a series of international workshops. These workshops have established a nomenclature for leukocyte surface antigens. Each characterized antigen is given a 'CD' number, and there are currently 168 CDs.

2.1 A brief, boring but necessary discourse on nomenclature

The term CD stood initially for cluster of differentiation; the 'cluster' referring to the statistical procedure that grouped together antibodies with similar reactivity when tested against a large panel of cells. The term cluster has led to some confusion (it does not mean that the molecule occurs on the cell in a 'cluster' of molecules); the term CD is sometimes said to stand for cluster determinant. It is best to think of it simply as CD, not short for anything, but indicating that the molecule, and the antibodies against it, have been subjected to the rigorous multi-laboratory studies of the international workshops on Human Leukocyte Differentiation Antigens (HLDA).

A further source of confusion – does CD identify the antigen or the antibody? Originally the intention was to describe antibodies which were clustered on the basis of similar reactivity. At that time, for many of the antibodies the eliciting antigen was not known; it was distinctly possible that a CD would end up containing antibodies against two or more unrelated antigens, which were generally coexpressed. Thus initially CD identified the antibodies. Gradually, and without any specific decision to that effect, CD has come to identify the antigen, the molecule detected by the clustered antibodies. This makes sense, since it is generally the molecule that is the subject of study; the antibody is no more than a tool for identifying the molecule. Nevertheless, the use of CD to describe an antibody is still important to indicate that this particular antibody has been through the workshop process – there have been numerous instances of antibodies described as belonging to a particular CD on the basis of the originator's own data which have turned out, upon Workshop analysis, to be against something else.

In summary the use of the term CD to describe the molecule, and antibodies against it, may seem chaotic but in practise it works well, and the context will usually make it clear whether the antibody or the antigen is under discussion. The term 'anti-CDxx' to describe an antibody is useful to avoid confusion.

2.2 The distribution of molecules among cell types

Some molecules are characteristic of specific cell types. The T cell receptor is the *sine qua non* of the T cell; immunoglobulin is the defining characteristic of a B lymphocyte. Even in such relatively straightforward instances there are complicating factors; immunoglobulin is found as a soluble protein in the serum and tissues, and it binds to many cells. Thus it is important to know that immunoglobulin is actually made by a cell before we can be sure it is a B cell. On the other hand, cells of the B cell lineage express readily-detectable immunoglobulin on their surface during a restricted part of their life cycle, and failure to detect immunoglobulin by cell surface staining is consistent with a cell either being completely unrelated to the B lineage, or a cell of the B lineage at a particular stage in activation or differentiation when immunoglobulin is not expressed on the surface.

Many molecules serve as useful markers of groups of cells but with a complex relationship to cell type. CD45 identifies a family of molecules which include a molecule known as the leukocyte-common antigen. All leukocytes express CD45 in one form or another; and, as far as is known, all cells expressing CD45 are leukocytes. CD45 is found in a number of molecular isoforms – molecular variants. The gene coding for CD45 includes three additional exons that may be spliced in or not, so that the CD45 protein can exist in a number of splice isoforms. In addition, the molecule may be variably glycosylated, leading to additional heterogeneity. An antibody (UCHL-1), which reacts with the form of the molecule which lacks any of the additional splice inserts (CD45RO), reacts with a proportion of T lymphocytes, as well as some myeloid cells. A number of antibodies classified as CD45RA react with a different sub-population of T lymphocytes (as well as B cell as some myeloid cells). By and large, T cells which express high levels of CD45RO do not express high levels of CD45RA. On the basis of a large body of experimental data, it has been concluded that T cells initially express CD45RA, but activation leads to a gradual loss of CD45RA and its replacement with CD45RO. CD45RO-positive T cells are therefore cells that have previously been activated, and are often referred to as memory cells.

This is a very useful distinction, with a great deal of relevance to T cell function. But we must remember that it is not as clear-cut as the statement: "A cell expressing T cell receptor is a T cell". The relationship between CD45 isoform and T cell memory is more complex for a number of reasons. First, there is a numerically, and perhaps functionally significant population of T cells which express both CD45RA and RO. Second, the definition of a memory T cell is conceptually complex, and we have to avoid the trap of using a simple marker to mask the complexity of the concept. Third, what experimental studies show is that the CD45RO population include cells that might reasonably be called memory cells; the experiments have not, at least as yet, shown that every CD45RO-positive cell has memory function. So to refer to CD45RO-positive cells as memory cells is an extrapolation beyond our knowledge.

This example has been discussed in some detail to illustrate the complexity of the relationship between cell phenotype and function. Providing these limitations are borne in mind, cell phenotype studies can be enormously useful in understanding cell function. Assessment of cell phenotype has become an important part of the clinical laboratory assessment of patients with immunological malfunction, including immune deficiency, autoimmune disease and allergy, as well as patients being immunosuppressed to prevent rejection of organ transplants.

3. Cell markers: identification and enumeration of specific cell types

This section will deal with methods for the analysis of cells in suspension. Analysis of tissue sections will be discussed in a later section.

The availability of antibodies against many cell surface molecules (CD1 to CD168 and many other markers not included in the CD classification) provides a powerful analytical resource, but how do we use it? Antibodies are not directly visible, and they must be rendered visible. By far the most useful approach to visualizing antibody binding on cells in suspension is fluorescence – the attachment to the antibody of a fluorescent dye. Antibodies may be linked to enzymes, which are in turn detected by chromogenic substrates – substrates which are not themselves necessarily colored but which, after being acted on by the enzyme, give a colored product. These are widely used in tissue section staining and will be described in the appropriate section. An alternative approach is to link a radioactive isotope to the antibody, and detect the radioactivity. Radioisotopic methods are capable of great sensitivity (detecting small numbers of antibody molecules and hence small numbers of antigen molecules) but are increasingly out of favor because of the safety implications of working with radioactivity; they also lack the analytical power of fluorescence coupled with flow methods of analysis (see below).

3.1 Fluorescence

Some substances absorb light and re-emit it at a higher wavelength. This phenomenon is called fluorescence. The reason for the change in wavelength is that part of the absorbed light energy is converted to other forms of energy, so that when the photons are re-emitted they have lower energy than the absorbed photons; energy and wavelength are inversely correlated, so the emitted light is always of a higher wavelength. The change in wavelength is constant for a given fluorescent substance (fluorophore, or fluorochrome), and is called the Stokes shift.

If we stain cells with an antibody to which has been coupled a non-fluorescent dye, we can readily detect cells which have bound the antibody. This can be done very effectively using a microscope, and it is possible to automate the process of detection using video image analysis. The optical set-up for detecting fluorescence is more complex, requiring filters to separate the incident wavelength from the emitted wavelength. Fluorescence has very considerable advantages which out-weigh the need for more complex equipment. First, fluorescence is capable of very high sensitivity, matching that of radioisotopic methods and exceeding that of methods based on dyes which simply absorb light. Second, the light emission by a fluorescent compound allows detection of the signal at angles other than the straight-through, 180° angle. In microscopy this allows the design of epi-illumination systems, where the light is directed at the sample from above and the emitted light is measured after coming back up the same path. The wavelength change characteristic of fluorescence allows the use of optical filters to select for the fluorescent signal and reject scattered light of the incident wavelength. The advantage of epi-illumination and optical separation of the emitted from the incident light is an improvement in contrast.

3.2 Flow cytometry

Cells in suspension may be stained and deposited on a microscope slide for examination in the microscope. Alternatively, they may be analyzed in suspension, by causing them to flow through an optical system that illuminates them and analyzes the emitted signals. This technology is known as flow cytometry, occasionally flow microfluorimetry and, commonly but inappropriately, FACS analysis. The use of the latter term is inappropriate because FACS is a trade name and not all instruments are made by the same manufacturer, and because FACS stands for fluorescence-activated cell sorting – the 'sorting' referring to the separation of cells (which will be discussed later).

Flow cytometry is immensely powerful because the combination of multiple antibodies with different fluorochromes, together with physical parameters which can be measured simultaneously, allows the analysis of multiple (five easily, nine in specialized instruments) parameters, on a cell-by-cell basis to build up a detailed analytical profile of a cell mixture.

The configuration of a typical flow cytometer is illustrated schematically in *Figure 6.1a*, whilst *Figure 6.1b* shows a photograph of the sorting section of a cell sorter. Cells in suspension are forced through a narrow channel and a separately-pressurized stream of buffer ('sheath fluid') compresses the cell stream so that cells flow in single file through a light beam, usually a laser beam. As each cell passes through the beam, a number of different light signals can be recorded. The cell scatters light in all directions, but the intensity of the scattered signal in a forward direction (low angle scatter or forward scatter) is approximately proportional to cell size, while the intensity of the scatter signal at 90° (side scatter) is proportional to a summation of physical properties which may best be described as structuredness, or complexity. A cell with a rough surface membrane will scatter more intensely at 90° than a cell with a smoother membrane. A cell with many complex intracellular organelles (mitochondria, lysosomes, etc.) will give a larger side-scatter signal than a cell with fewer intracellular organelles. Side-scatter and forward scatter together allow reliable identification of distinct populations such as platelets, red cells, lymphocytes, granulocytes and monocytes in a mixture.

The use of fluorochrome-labeled antibodies allows specific identification of cell type. Combination of different antibodies with different fluorochromes allows the simultaneous identification of multiple cell types, the identification of cell subpopulations, or the analysis of phenotype of cells belonging to particular populations. This multiparameter capability is the real power of fluorescence flow cytometry, and will be illustrated with a few examples.

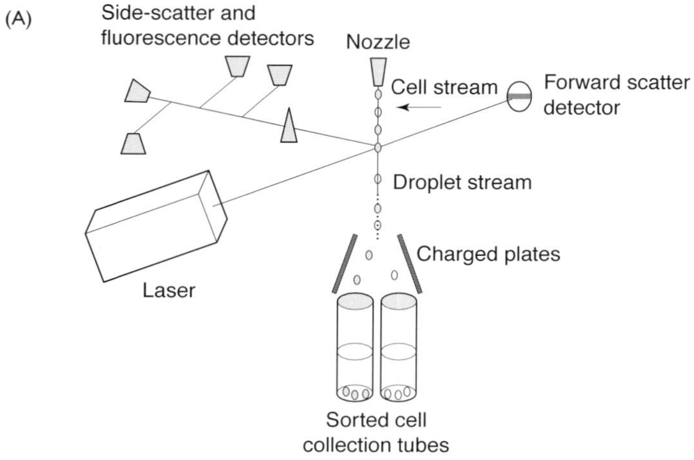

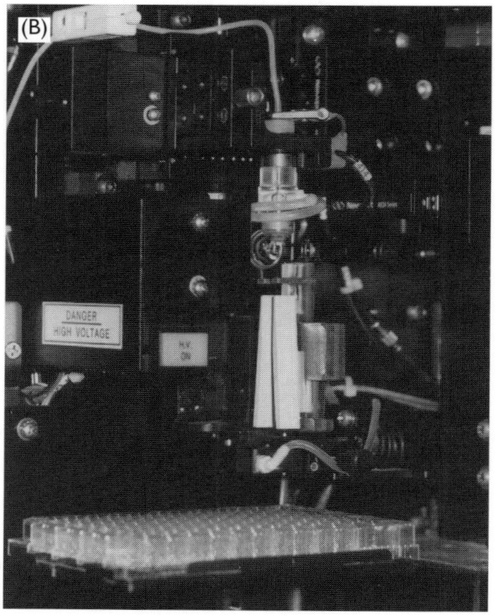

Figure 6.1

(A) Diagrammatic representation of a flow cytometer/fluorescence-activated cell sorter. (B) Photograph of cell sorting assembly of fluorescence-activated cell sorter. The stream of cells can be seen emerging from the nozzle, and passing between the charged plates (see Fig.6.1a). The sorter is set up to sort single cells into wells of a microtiter tray.

In *Figure 6.2* a sample of blood is analyzed. The two scatter parameters allow the identification of the lymphocyte population, and the instrument can be instructed to analyze the fluorescence of these cells only. CD3, a component of the T cell receptor, is a reliable marker for T cells, and can be used to positively identify T cells. CD19 is a reliable marker for B cells, and a combination of CD19 and CD3 with different fluorochromes allows the identification of three populations, T cells, B cells and cells which are neither T nor B cells (*Figure 6.3*). We would not expect to find any cells

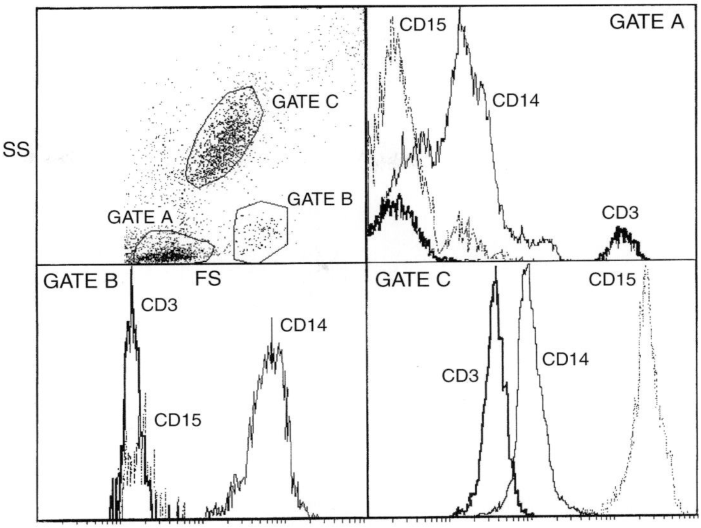

Figure 6.2

Analysis of blood cells. The top left box shows side-scatter (SS) plotted against forward scatter (FS), with populations selected in 'gates' A (lymphocytes), B (monocytes and blast cells) and C (polymorphonuclear cells). The remaining panels show staining with CD3 (T lymphocyte marker), CD14 (monocyte marker) and CD15 (polymorph marker) on the cells in gates A, B and C. Gate A contains T cells (bright positive for CD3 and non-T lymphocytes (negative for CD3), and the majority of cells show weak staining with CD14 and very weak staining for CD15. Gate A contains some monocytes, evident from the small population of CD14 brightly positive cells. Gate B contains cells uniformly bright for CD14 and much weaker for CD3 or CD15; Gate C contains cells very bright for CD15, weak for CD14 and weaker still for CD3.

expressing both CD3 and CD19. On the other hand, we would expect the majority of cells expressing CD4, a T cell subset marker, to also express CD3, since CD3 is present on all T cells (*Figure 6.4*).

Two-color fluorescence allows the identification of the CD4 subset of T cells, using CD4/CD3 dual labeling. If we want to know what proportion of CD4 T cells are activated, we can add a third fluorochrome attached to an activation marker (CD25 in this case) and identify cells which coexpress CD3, CD4, and CD25.

Most commonly available instruments will provide data on two scatter parameters and two fluorochromes; the standard instruments being manufactured today provide a third fluorescence parameter. Analysis of more than three fluorescence parameters (more than five parameters altogether) requires more sophisticated instrumentation but the principles are essentially the same.

3.3 Fluorochromes and optical systems

The most widely used light-source in cytometers currently is the argon-ion laser. Tunable argon-ion lasers are capable of providing excitation at a range of wavelengths, allowing the use of a variety of fluorochromes. However, these tunable lasers are expensive to buy and to run, requiring water-

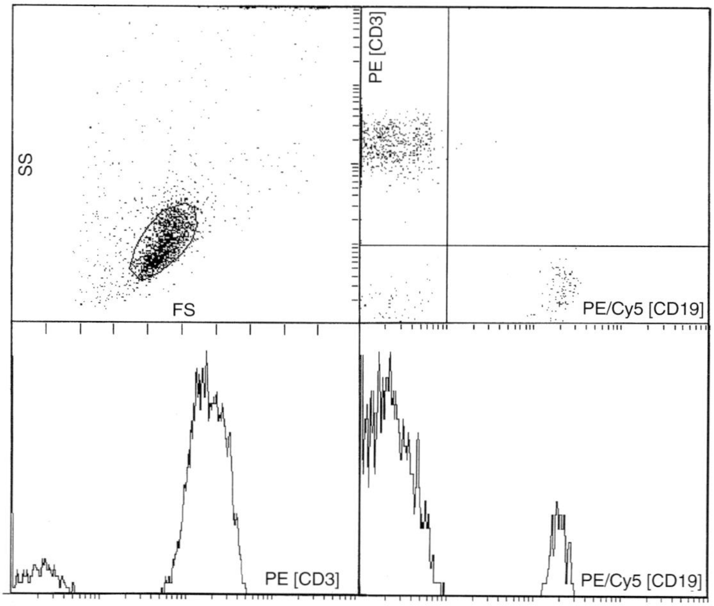

Figure 6.3

Two-color analysis of lymphocyte fraction. Top left: dual scatter parameters (see Figure 6.2 *caption for explanation). Top right: two-color analysis with CD3 and CD19. Lower traces: individual CD3 and CD19 staining.*

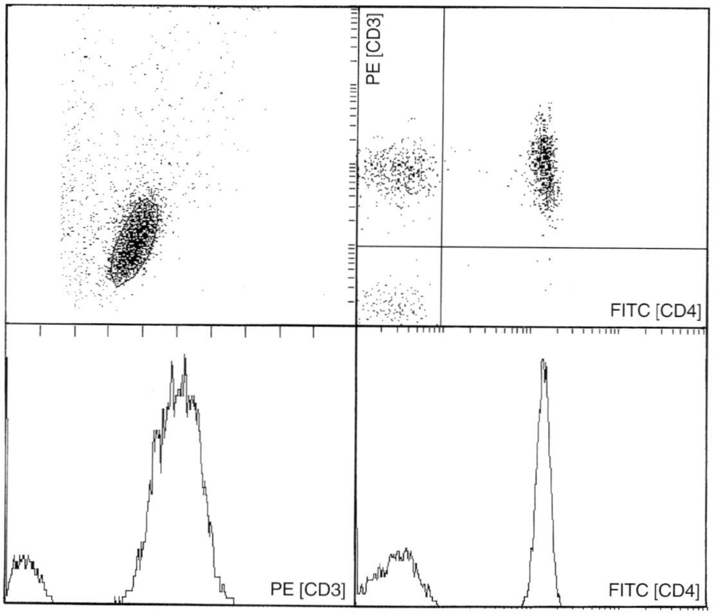

Figure 6.4

Two-color analysis of lymphocyte fraction. Top left: dual scatter parameters (see Figure 6.2 *caption for explanation). Top right: two-color analysis with CD3 and CD4. Lower traces: individual CD3 and CD4 staining.*

cooling. A smaller, air-cooled argon-ion laser is available at relatively low cost, but the only wavelength at which it emits significant power is 488 nm, and these lasers are provided as fixed-wavelength (nontunable) 488 nm lasers, usually with a maximum power of 15 mW.

The selection of the 488 nm argon-ion laser as the standard light source governs the selection of suitable dyes, which must absorb 488 nm light strongly. The most widely-used dye is fluorescein, which absorbs strongly at 488 nm and can readily be prepared in chemical forms which can easily be conjugated to protein. Fluorescein is usually the dye used in single-color fluorescence analysis, but in multiparameter analysis we need additional dyes, which can also be excited at 488 nm but which emit at wavelengths well-separated from the fluorescein emission.

Now we have to start making compromises, because most of the other dyes available have absorption maxima significantly away from 488 nm, and have emission spectra with significant overlap with that of fluorescein. In practice, as long as a dye absorbs significantly at 488 nm it matters not that it can absorb better at a different wavelength. The consequences of overlapping emission spectra are minimized in part by using filters to collect only part of the emission spectrum (*Figure 6.5*), and any residual overlap can be corrected for using electronic means (to be discussed in detail below).

It is worth pointing out that fluorescein is not always the dye of choice. Phycoerythrin (PE) gives a much stronger signal, so that for applications where sensitivity is important phycoerythrin is the dye of choice. Spectral overlap between phycoerythrin and phycoerythrin-Cy5 'tandem' dyes is less than that between fluorescein and phycoerythrin, so that the PE/PE-Cy5 combination offers some advantages over the PE-fluorescein combination.

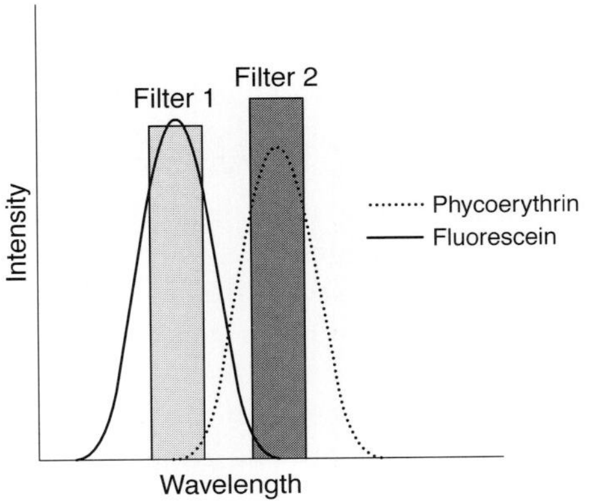

Figure 6.5

Emission spectra of two fluorescent dyes, fluorescein and phycoerythrin. The dyes emit at different wavelengths (the wavelength difference between the peaks is the Stokes' shift) but they overlap to some degree. The overlap can be reduced by using narrow-band filters, but there remains some phycoerythrin signal in the fluorescein channel, and the long 'tail' of the fluorescein spectrum extends significantly into the phycoerythrin channel. These spectral overlaps can give rise to incorrect data and have to be removed by electronic compensation of the measured signals.

PE and PE-Cy5 are excited better at 542 nm than at 488 nm, so that there is a rationale for a system based on a solid-state YAG laser emitting at 542 nm used in combination with PE-based dyes, instead of the current 488 nm-based system. However, for the foreseeable future, most instruments are restricted to 488 nm and are nevertheless very powerful, with the available dyes.

3.4 Staining methods

Staining of cell membrane antigens with antibody can be performed by direct immunofluorescence or by indirect immunofluorescence. In direct immunofluorescence an antibody against the molecule of interest is conjugated directly to fluorophore. Staining consists of a single step, followed by washing away excess reagent. Several variants of indirect immunofluorescence may be used; in all of them antibody against the antigen of interest is *not* directly conjugated to fluorophore, but is in turn detected by a fluorophore-conjugated second-step reagent (see *Chapter 5*). Indirect procedures require at least two reagent binding steps, separated by washes.

The advantage of direct staining is speed and simplicity, if the directly conjugated reagents are available. If they are not, fluorophore-conjugation of antibody can be carried out by methods well within the capability of a typical research laboratory, but the procedures, and the need for extensive quality control justify consideration of indirect methods. Indirect staining methods are more time-consuming and somewhat more complex than direct immunofluorescence; the complexity brings with it a greater risk of nonspecific binding that may complicate interpretation. The major attraction of indirect methods is their suitability for use with unpurified antibodies, including sera, ascites fluids and hybridoma supernatants, as well as tagged engineered antibodies. The same method and reagent set can be used to examine a large number of different antibodies by indirect immunofluorescence. It is common in multicolor analysis to combine direct with indirect procedures.

3.5 Nonspecific staining and autofluorescence

The most intractable problem in immunofluorescence is nonspecific fluorescence, which confounds interpretation and reduces sensitivity. There are several possible causes of nonspecific fluorescence, and generally several will occur together, so that recognizing and reducing nonspecific fluorescence is an important skill.

Cells contain a variety of molecules that fluoresce, and so will emit a fluorescence signal without the addition of fluorochromes. This is known as autofluorescence. Intensities of autofluorescence vary according to the cell type, but generally the intensity of autofluorescence is much lower than the intensities achieved with fluorochrome-labeled antibodies. To determine the level of autofluorescence, run a control with no added reagents, and compare it with a positively-stained sample. If autofluorescence is a significant problem it may be worth experimenting with different laser-dye combinations, since cellular autofluorescence is generally less in the orange-red part of the spectrum (PE emission) than in the green (fluorescein emission).

While autofluorescence is generally not a significant problem, nonspecific binding of reagents to cells is a frequent and unpredictable source of trouble. There are two major and distinct causes for nonspecific binding. The reagents used in the detection sequence may cross-react with a molecule expressed on the target cells. For example, in indirect immunofluorescence using mouse monoclonal anti-rat CD3, the antimouse Ig used to detect the monoclonal antibody is very likely to cross-react strongly with rat Ig. This means that rat B lymphocytes, which do not express CD3 but do express Ig, will be stained. Whilst this cross-reactivity is to be expected, since the anti-mouse Ig is generally made in sheep, goat or horse, all species well-removed from the rodents which will see mouse and rat Ig as very similar, more distant cross-reactivities can also cause problems. Anti-mouse Ig cross-reacts to a small extent with human Ig and may give nonspecific staining of human B cells, especially in high sensitivity procedures.

Cross-reactivity, where the cross-reacting antigen is usually immunoglobulin, can be avoided by using direct staining procedures, removing the need to use anti-Ig reagents. If this is not possible, cross-reactivity may be reduced by careful choice of reagents, and by absorption if necessary. In the above example of staining rat cells with mouse monoclonal antibodies, a rat-anti-mouse Ig would not cross react significantly with rat Ig.

The other major source of nonspecific binding derives from the tendency of proteins, including antibodies, to bind to structures on cells other than the specific antigen they recognize. This binding may be due to an identifiable ligand/receptor interaction or may be simply nonspecific binding through weak protein–protein interactions. The latter can usually be minimized by thorough washing of cells and by inclusion of protein in the incubation and wash buffers. The receptor/ligand interaction which causes most nonspecific immunofluorescence is the interaction of the Fc segment of antibody with Fc receptors on cells.

There are three classes of Fc receptors for IgG, as well as known receptors for IgE and IgA, and probable receptors for IgM. These Fc receptors are widely distributed within and outside the immune system. They differ in affinity for Ig, with two of the IgG receptors having low affinity for monomeric IgG but high affinity for aggregated or complexed IgG. The broad distribution and complexity makes it difficult to predict precisely where difficulties are likely to be encountered with Fc mediated nonspecific binding, but generally B cells and monocytes show stronger non-specific binding than T cells, and problems are more likely to be encountered with Ig which has been frozen and thawed or chemically modified, both of which can lead to partial denaturation and aggregation. In direct immunofluorescence the monoclonal antibody itself may bind through Fc interactions; in indirect methods the monoclonal antibody or any of the detection reagents may bind. The presence of Fc receptors may cause the cells to retain Ig derived from the serum they were originally bathed in. This should not cause non-specific signals, unless the detection reagent cross-reacts with this species of IgG.

A number of approaches to reducing Fc mediated binding may be tried; it is difficult to predict which one will work best in a particular situation.

Centrifuging reagents to remove larger aggregates may be useful. Preincubating cells in normal serum may block Fc receptors; the species of serum to be used must be selected to avoid cross-reactivity. If possible the same species as that used to make the major detection antibody should be used, reducing the chance of cross-reactivity. Avian Ig does not bind well to mammalian Fc receptors, so that chicken sera are useful reagents in reducing Fc-mediated background.

The final word on nonspecific binding is that many studies can be done without encountering problems, but it is important to recognize and deal with non-specific binding when it occurs. Inclusion of appropriate controls (*Figure 6.6*) helps to detect and assess the severity of non-specific binding.

3.6 Intracellular antigens

Whilst the majority of antibody based flow cytometric studies have focused on molecules expressed on the outer face of the cell membrane, there are vitally interesting changes going on inside the cell. Studies on intracellular antigens are much more difficult than studies on surface antigens, because the cell must be permeabilized to allow the antibody in yet must retain the antigen of interest. While methods to achieve this have been available for some years they were difficult to reproduce. In recent years, stimulated by an interest in analyzing the intracellular content of cytokines particularly in helper T cells, there has been a refinement of technique which has precipitated an avalanche of studies on intracellular antigen staining.

This technology is still not free of difficulty, but it can answer very interesting questions – for example what cells respond to a specific antigenic stimulus such as a bacterial antigen or an allergen, and what is the nature of that response.

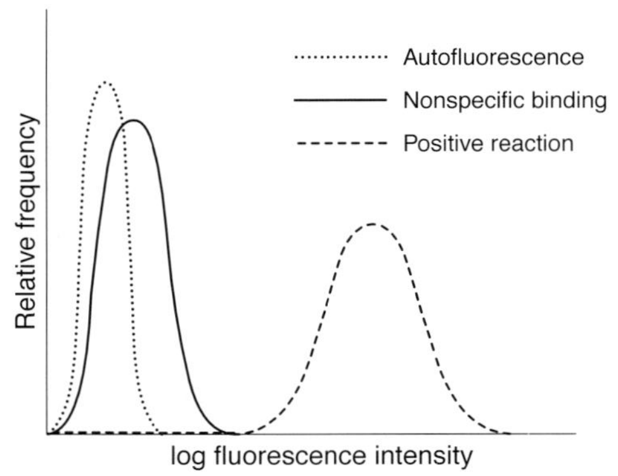

Figure 6.6

Fluorescence histograms obtained with unstained cells, representing autofluorescence; cells stained with reagents against an antigen absent from the cells, representing nonspecific binding, and cells stained with an antibody against an antigen present at high concentration on the majority of cells.

3.7 Nonantibody parameters

Apart from the two light-scatter parameters, flow cytometry can be used to measure a number of other cellular properties using methods independent of antibodies. These are outside the scope of this book, but they can all be combined with antibodies in multiparameter assays and the reader should be aware of the power of the technology.

Dyes which cannot pass an intact cell membrane but can pass through a damaged membrane are used to distinguish live from dead cells. It is often convenient to combine such a dye with immunofluorescence in order to focus the analysis on live cells. Dyes which bind DNA or RNA quantitatively can be used to label cells according to their cell-cycle stage. Dyes that bind to the membrane can be used to measure cell surface area; as cells divide these dyes are shared by the daughter cells and the staining intensity thus indicates the number of cell divisions that have occurred since labeling; a similar technique which loads cells with a fluorescein derivative may be used to relate function to the number of cell divisions.

Calcium-binding dyes can be used to detect calcium ion fluxes that accompany cellular processes; similarly probes for internal pH and for membrane potential can be used to measure metabolic processes. A variety of flow cytometric methods are available for the detection of cell apoptosis. Fluorochrome-labelled DNA or RNA probes can be used for fluorescence-based *in situ* hybridization (FISH).

All of these methods can be combined with antibody based markers to focus the analysis on a particular cell type or subpopulation.

4. Antibody-based cell separation

If an antibody can be used to identify a cell type, it can in principle be used as a 'handle' to isolate that cell type. There are several antibody-based cell methods, and each can be carried out in positive selection or negative selection modes. In positive selection the cells of interest are stained by a monoclonal antibody specific for that population. Positive selection methods are capable of giving high purity (typically 95–98%). The principal disadvantage is that antibodies that bind cells frequently activate them. If the cells are required in their native state, negative selection, where all other cells are coated with antibody and removed, is suitable. However, it is more difficult to achieve high purity by negative selection. If for example we are trying to isolate T cells from blood, we must have antibodies against all cells that are not T cells, not just the major populations. Separation of antibody-coated cells is never perfect, and a proportion of cells that bind the antigen will not bind enough, or will for some other reason slip through the isolation procedure. In positive selection, these cells will reduce the yield, but not the purity – in negative selection they will reduce purity. On the other hand, cells which do not express the antigen but bind antibody non-specifically will contaminate the purified population in positive selection, but not in negative selection.

Techniques for antibody-specified separation can best be divided into fluorescence-activated cell sorting and affinity-based methods, because there is a significant difference in principle between these two categories.

Affinity-based methods include the use of magnetic beads and antibody-coated surfaces such as cell-culture dishes or gel particles. The bead or surface is coated with antibody against the cell surface antigen which forms the basis of the separation or, by analogy with indirect immunofluorescence staining methods, the cell is coated with the antibody and the bead or surface with an anti-immunoglobulin, or avidin if the antibody is biotinylated.

The difference in principle between fluorescence-activated cell sorting and the affinity based methods is important and seems not to be widely appreciated. In fluorescence activated cell sorting the antibody acts as a label to identify the cells; the physical separation is based on a drop-charging system with the charged droplets being separated in an electrostatic field. As long as antibody binding is strong enough to identify the population of interest, the separation does not depend on antibody binding to be strong enough to actually achieve the separation. Contrast this with the use of magnetic beads or 'panning' on an antibody-coated surface. The binding of the cells by the antibody is what actually mediates the separation. The binding must be strong enough to withstand shear forces during multiple washes and during the separation itself. For such a method to work the antigen should be present at high concentration on the cell surface (typically 20 000 copies per cell or more); the antigen should not be easily shed from the cell, the antibody should have a high affinity for antigen and particularly a slow dissociation rate. These properties can also influence fluorescence-based sorting, since there must be enough antibody on the cell surface to distinguish positive from negative cells, but they are less critical.

These considerations highlight one major distinction between fluorescence-based sorting and affinity methods. The other is that fluorescence based sorting separates one cell at a time. High throughput rates can be achieved, but nevertheless sorting is relatively slow and suited to separation of small numbers of cells, whereas the affinity-based methods are capable of being scaled up to any desired level. The choice between sorting and affinity based methods is thus dictated by the needs of the experiment and the availability of suitable reagents; the methods are complementary and are often used in tandem (for example panning or magnetic beads to enrich a major population, followed by sorting to isolate a specific cell type).

Flow sorting has a major capability which the other methods lack: the ability to separate cells on the basis of multiple parameters simultaneously. For example if we want to isolate from blood the subset of CD4-positive T cells that express CD25 we can do that by sorting using two scatter parameters to define the lymphocyte population, CD4 linked to fluorescein and CD25 detected with biotinylated antibody and PE-streptavidin.

It is essential to determine purity critically – there are too many publications simply stating that 'cells were purified on the basis of X'. Purity can vary day by day using ostensibly the same procedure, and purity must be determined on the actual preparation being used, or at the very least consistency of purity must be demonstrated. The parameters used to demonstrate purity should be distinct from those used to effect the separation. To show that T cells purified with a CD3 antibody contain 98% CD3-positive cells is not particularly useful – if the CD3 antibody preparation was aggregated and bound to monocytes and B cells through Fc receptors they would be copurified, and would show up as CD3-positive. A demonstration that 98% of the cells expressed either CD4 or CD8, and less than 1% expressed CD19 (a B cell marker) or CD14 (a monocyte marker) would be much more convincing.

5. Antibody-based cell destruction or agglutination

Killing a subset of cells based on their expression of a particular antigen may be seen as another cell separation procedure. Cell killing is usually achieved on the basis of complement fixation. Complement is a series of proteins found in the serum which bind to antibody on cells and initiate an enzymatic reaction cascade which culminates in the insertion of holes in the cell membrane. Not all antibodies bind complement, but IgM and some IgG subclasses bind complement effectively. There is no need for the antibody and complement to be from the same species, and rabbit complement is widely used with mouse monoclonal antibodies.

Complement-mediated cytotoxicity is not widely used, having been largely displaced by the methods described in the last section. It is difficult to achieve 100% kill of the target population, and some of the products of the complement cascade will activate other cells. Nevertheless there are some situations where complement-mediated killing is still useful. A related method uses antibody, usually IgM, to agglutinate cells which may then be removed by centrifugation or simply by allowing the clumps to settle. Again, this 'old-fashioned' method is not widely used but can be powerful in some situations – we have for example found it useful in removing red cell precursors which contaminate mononuclear cell populations isolated from cold blood.

6. Analysis of function

Monoclonal antibodies can be applied to the study of cell function in a number of ways. Antibodies can be used, as described in previous sections, to purify, remove or destroy sub-populations of cells and assess their function or their contribution to a particular function. In a classic example widely used in studies on the mechanisms of transplant rejection, injection of a cell population into an animal mediates a function – graft rejection, or graft tolerance for example. To assess the contributions of various subpopulations, for example CD4 cells, to this phenomenon, animals are injected with the whole population and with the population after treatment with anti-CD4 antibody and complement, to destroy CD4 cells.

Antibodies against cell-surface molecules frequently mediate signals to the cell, initiating activation, proliferation, or apoptosis. It is often assumed that such 'agonistic antibodies' mimic the effect of the physiological ligand. Whilst this is an insecure assumption, cell activation by antibodies does provide an in vitro model for studies of activation and its control.

The result of cell activation often includes the expression of specific gene products on the cell surface; for example cytokine receptors and molecules involved in intercellular interactions. The use of antibodies to examine changes in cell surface phenotype as a result of *in vitro* or *in vivo* activation has provided a rich source of information on cell activation. Extension of this approach to cytoplasmic molecules, such as cytokines or markers of proliferation currently promises to provide a clearer picture of immunological mechanisms.

7. Tissue analysis

Flow cytometry provides a powerful analytical approach, thanks to its precision and capacity to measure several properties simultaneously on each cell of a population. Nevertheless, it has two major limitations. The first is that important topographical information is lost when a tissue is converted into a single-cell suspension – the positional relationships between cells of different type and function provides strong clues on mechanism. The second limitation of the cell-suspension approach is that not all tissues can be converted into suspensions of well behaved (roughly spherical, nonadhering) single cells without significant damage. This is the major reason that flow cytometry has been largely restricted to studies of the immune system. Cells of the nervous system depend on their complex shape for their function; cells of many tissues cannot be obtained in suspension without the use of proteolytic enzymes, which will affect many of their surface properties.

Consequently, immunohistology, which predates flow cytometry, remains an important technology and has been strengthened by the advent of monoclonal antibodies.

Immunohistology, or immunohistochemistry (the names can be used interchangeably, although histochemistry originally referred to the use of chemical reactions to visualize tissue components), simply means the use of antibodies in the study of tissue. The tissue can be either fixed and embedded in paraffin or polymeric material for sectioning, or cut from blocks of frozen tissue (referred to as cryostat material). Fixed/embedded material generally shows superior preservation of morphology, but many molecules are modified by the fixative and embedding material and may no longer be recognized by antibody. Cryostat sections are generally more likely to provide accurate data on expression of molecules.

Immunohistology has long played an important role in pathology, allowing the analysis of disease processes – for example distinguishing between a malignant and an inflammatory proliferation of lymphocytes. Immunohistology was well established in pathology before the advent of monoclonal antibodies, but now makes extensive use of the greater specificity and analytical power of monoclonal antibodies. Polyclonal reagents are more likely to react with fixed/embedded material, because the greater diversity of epitopes increases the probability of including epitopes that are resistant to fixation and embedding. Thus the change from polyclonal to monoclonal reagents has been accompanied by a change to cryostat material.

There are two major alternative methodologies to convert the binding of an antibody to a visible color reaction: enzymatic methods and fluorescence. Pathologists have generally preferred enzymatic methods because they allow counterstaining and visualization of staining in the context of clear morphology. Immunofluorescence generally allows greater sensitivity and contrast, but visualization of unstained material, and therefore the surrounding morphology, is poor compared with immunoenzymatic methods.

In summary, for any particular application the user must chose between cryostat and fixed/embedded sections, between monoclonal and polyclonal antibodies, between immunofluorescence and immunoenzymatic methods of visualization. To some extent the decisions are interrelated – immunofluorescence tends to give high nonspecific staining with embedded material; monoclonal antibodies often do not work with embedded material. As a general guide, if a monoclonal antibody is available it should be used in preference to a polyclonal antiserum because there is a lower risk on nonspecific staining; if a monoclonal antibody is selected this will tend to favor the use of cryostat sections. If seeing the stained cells in the context of surrounding, unstained material is important, enzymatic methods of visualization are to be preferred; if sensitivity and contrast between stained and unstained material is important fluorescence is likely to be more useful.

Many of the general principles discussed for fluorescence when used in flow cytometry apply also in fluorescence microscopy, although different dyes may be preferred – fluorescein is widely used, but phycoerythrin fades extremely rapidly and the cyanine dye Cy3 is preferred. Two-color immunofluorescence and immunoenzymatic staining methods have been used successfully, but are not routine as they are in flow cytometry.

Further Reading

Robinson, J.P. (ed) (1999) *Current Protocols in Cytometry.* John Wiley and Sons, New York.

Protocol 6.1

Direct immunofluorescence

Materials

Sample: whole blood in anticoagulant, mononuclear cell fraction or suspension of tissue cells

PBS/azide: Dulbecco's phosphate buffered saline or other isotonic buffer with added sodium azide at 0.02 M

Fluorochrome-labelled monoclonal antibodies as required, isotype control with the same fluorochrome and at the same concentration

Tubes to hold 3 ml and fit cytometer

Ice/water container

Refrigerated centrifuge with rotor capable of centrifuging up to 64 reaction tubes

Protocol

Keep cells cold throughout by standing the reaction tubes in melting ice and centrifuging at 4°C.

1. Prepare mononuclear cells from blood or tissue using Ficoll-hypaque. Suspend cells at 10^7 ml^{-1} in PBS/azide. Whole blood may be used; erythrocytes must be lyzed after staining.
2. Add monoclonal antibody as directed by the manufacturer (usually 5 μl). Mix gently, incubate on melting ice for 30 min.
3. Add 3 ml of cold PBS/azide and centrifuge at 200 **g** for 5 min. Remove the supernatant by gentle aspiration, being careful to remove as much of the liquid as possible without disturbing the cell pellet.
4. Resuspend the cells in 100–200 μl cold PBS/azide if flow cytometry is to be carried out on the same day; if analysis is to be delayed resuspend in 200 μl flow cytometry fixative. Add the directly conjugated monoclonal antibody.
5. Analyze by flow cytometry. Select cell population of interest by gating on forward and side-scatter parameters and print out fluorescence intensity histograms (see *Figures 6.2, 6.3* and *6.4* for examples).

Notes

1. Sodium azide reacts with copper pipes to form an explosive compound. Waste containing azide should be disposed of in plastic plumbing; check with Institutional Safety Officer.

2. The use of an isotype-matched negative control is essential, but does not guarantee that staining is specific, because nonspecific binding is affected by the fluorochrome conjugation and by aggregation or denaturation during purification or storage, so that no two preparations are quite the same.
3. Indirect immunofluorescence and procedures involving both direct and indirect immunofluorescence are more complex but follow the same principle – see *Further Reading* for detailed protocols.

The Basics

Index

Adjuvant, 21–22, 35
  complete Freund's, xiv, 21–22
  Gerbu, 22, 35
  incomplete Freund's, xiv, 21–22
Affinity, xiii, 48, 54–55
  chromatography, xiii, 89–90, 95–96
  maturation, xiii, 1, 65
Agglutination, 141
Antibody
  as agonist, 127
  chimeric, 51–52
  clinical applications, 45–46, 47
  diversity, 1
  engineering, 15
  humanized, 51–52
  IgA, xv, 5
  IgG, xv, 5, 103, 105
  IgM, xv, 5, 103, 105
  immunogenicity, 46
  mutation, xvi, 1
  polyclonal, xvi, 8, 10–11
  selection, xvi, 1
  specificity, 1
  structure, 2–5
  therapeutic applications, 13, 45, 47
Antigen identification, 12
  localization, 12
  quantitation, 13
  purification, 13
Ascitic fluid, 27
Autofluorescence, 136–138
Avidity, xiii, 48–49

B lymphocyte xiii, 5, 6, 132
  memory, xv, 6
  Naïve, xv, 6
  precursors (progenitors) xiii, 6
Bacterial infection, diagnosis, 112–121
Bacteriology, 110–121

Calcium, intracellular, 139
Cancer, 45
CD (cluster of differentiation) antigens, 128, 130
  CD3, 132, 141
  CD4, 133, 140–141
  CD8, 141
  CD14, 141
  CD19, 132
  CD25, 133, 140
  CD45, 129
  CD45R0, 129
  CD45RA, 129
Cell
  analysis, 127–145
  cycle, 139
  destruction, 141
  function, 127, 141–142
  markers, *see* Cell membrane antigens
  membrane antigens, 127–145
  separation, 139–141
    affinity-based, 139–141
Chlamydia, 108, 110
Cloning, xiv, 26, 39
Complement, xiv, 3–5, 120
Conditioned medium, xiv, 25
Cryopreservation, 26, 40–41
Cytomegalovirus, 107–108
Cytotoxicity, 141

Diagnosis
  bacterial infection, 112–121, 124–126
  fungal infection, 121–122
  infection, 102–123
  parasitic infection, 121–122
  viral infection, 106–108
DNA, analysis, 139

ELISA, xiv, 32–33, 78, 83–86, 103
Enzyme activity, 87–89
Epitope, xiv, 86–87

Fc receptors, 137–138
Fetal calf serum, 19

Flow cytometry, 131–139, 118–119
  optical systems, 133–6
Fluorochromes, 133–134
Fluorescein, 135
Fluorescence, 130–131, 143
  in situ hybridization (FISH), 139
Fluorescence-activated cell sorting, 139–141
Fungal infection, 121–122
Fusion, *see* Hybridoma
  standard protocol, 36–38

Gene libraries, 15
Growth factor receptor, 127

HAMA (human anti-mouse antibody response), 51–52
Human immunodeficiency virus (HIV), 101, 104
Human Leukocyte Differentiation Antigen workshops, 128
Hybridoma, xv, 17–43
  screening and testing, 26–27, 32–33
  storage and quality control, 30–31

Immunization, 21–23, 35
  conjugation of antigen to carrier, 34
Immunoaffinity chromatography, 89–90, 95–96
Immunochemistry, 81
Immunoenzymatic methods, 108, 143
Immunofluorescence, 106–107, 110–112, 117–118
  direct, 144–145
  staining methods, 136
Immunoglobulin, *see also* Antibody
  C domain, xiii, 3
  CDR, xiv, 46
  constant region, 3
  Fab, xiv, 50–51,
    library in phage, 67–78
    purification, 79
  Fc, xiv, 3
  Fv, 46
  isotypes, 4, 5
  structure, 2
  V region, 6
Immunohistochemistry, 116, 142–143
Immunohistology, 122, 142–143
Immuno-organelle assay, 93
Immunoprecipitation, 92–93, 99–100
Infection, diagnosis, 102–123
Intracellular antigens, 138–139

Laser, argon ion, 135
Latex agglutination test, 124–126

Medium
  HAT, xiv, 24
  HT, 19, 24
  lysis, 20
  selection, 20
  serum free, 19

Monoclonal antibody
  definition xv, 9–11
  production – scale up, 27–29
  purification, 29
Mycoplasma, 27, 108, 109–110
Myeloma, 23

Nonspecific staining, 136–138

Parasitic infection, 121–122
PCR, xv, 36–38, 53–54
Phage display, xv, 57–65, 67–78
Phycoerythrin, 135, 143
Plasma cell, xvi, 5
Polyethylene glycol (PEG), 20
Protein A, xvi , 99–100
Protein G, xvi, 30, 42–43

Radiolabel
  biosynthesis, 92
  processing, 92
RNA, analysis, 139

ScFv, xvi, 46–50, 52–55
  expression, 55–57
  purification, 57
Serology, 103

T lymphocyte, xvi, 129, 132–133, 139
  memory, 129
  receptor, 129
Tandem dyes, 135
Tissue, analysis, 127, 142–143

Valency, xvi, 48–50
Viability, analysis, 139
Viral diagnosis, 106–108
Virus, 104–108
  antibodies against, 106–108

Western blotting, 91–92, 97–98